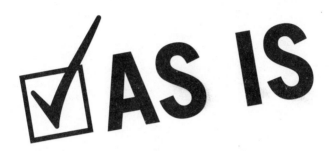

AS IS

CONFESSIONS
of a true
FATTY

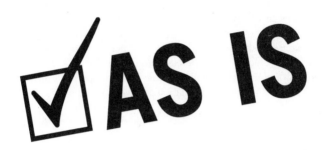

☑AS IS

CONFESSIONS
of a true
FATTY

LINDA MISLEH WAGNER

MisWags Press
7659 Mission Gorge Rd., Unit 68,
San Diego, CA 92120
lindamislehwagner@gmail.com

Printed in the United States of America

ISBN: 978-0-9906152-0-0 trade paperback

FIRST EDITION

Book design by GKS Creative

Library of Congress Cataloging-in-Publication Data

Wagner, Linda Misleh

As Is: Confessions of a True Fatty: the reasons and emotions behind weight gain, how to recognize what is causing binge eating, and what it takes to truly live a healthy life / Linda Misleh Wagner

HEA019000 HEALTH & FITNESS / Diet & Nutrition / Weight Loss
BIO026000 BIOGRAPHY & AUTOBIOGRAPHY / Personal Memoirs

DEDICATIONS

To My Daughter Nadia

You are a beautiful writer. You have always
encouraged and supported me, and you have
inspired me to go after my dreams.
I love you very much.

Mom

To My Husband, Bob,

If it wasn't for your love and your support and your
belief in making my dream become a reality, I could
not have done this body of work. I thank you for
allowing me to speak the truth and for giving me the
courage to face my realities with so much love.
I love you.

Linda

THE DANCE

She sits on the sidelines hoping someone will ask her to dance. The music pumps, the bodies on the dance floor gyrate. She looks at the women moving sensuously and teasingly with their male partners. She's envious of the women's bodies, all different yet each one beautiful and lean, with a flat stomach and long slender legs.

It's one of those warm summer evenings, so these beautiful women wear very little; they're obviously aware that they're hot and sexy with their bare backs and shoulders and arms, their short skirts or dresses. Although she is dressed very well—mainly in black, as usual—her back is completely covered, as are her arms and shoulders. Her blouse is long and tunic-style to cover her fatty belly and jelly-like thighs. The jeans under the blouse have an elasticized waist and tapered legs to give the illusion of skinny jeans on a not-so-skinny body. The only area she feels confident enough to show off is her cleavage. Nice big mammary glands—boobies, folks—are her one claim to body fame.

Despite her large figure, she has never been a sit-on-the-sidelines kind of gal; she is always the one who makes parties come alive. People love her because she's warm and caring and loving and funny. People open up to her and come to her to make their day better. She naturally exudes empathy and kindness. She makes them laugh. Despite her size she is considered beautiful by many people. "Exotic," "sexy," "graceful" are words used to describe her. Her dark, almond-shaped eyes attract people. "Bedroom eyes," men whisper to her.

But tonight, neither her eyes nor her personality are enticing a man to ask her to dance.

So she'll do the next best thing. She gets out of her chair and, swaying to the music, pulls her best friend to her feet. "Let's dance." And dance they do.

After four songs, both ladies decide to take a breather. As they make their way back to their table, people stop her to tell her how much they enjoyed her dancing. She is, after all, a very good dancer. Despite her size, this woman can MOVE.

So who is this woman? She is I, Linda Misleh Wagner. I am fifty-five years old, the mother of four children and grandmother of six. I've been married once, divorced once, and now married again. My second husband, Bob, is a wonderful man about whom I am absolutely insane, and he is crazy about me. He also loves to dance.

But if you've gotten the impression that along the way I've had to deal with weight problems, you're right.

It started early. I would describe my childhood self as "thick, vacuum-packed tuna," and myself for most of the rest of my life as "downright fat." Only for short bouts of time has my body weight been within normal limits—albeit the high end of normal limits. Five years to be exact, from age fourteen to age nineteen.

For the rest of my adult life I have been plagued by excess blubber. Oh, I've fought it. To say I've tried just about every diet, exercise video, and fast out there would not be an understatement. I own shelves, drawers and boxes full of DVDs, diet books, and exercise gear. I am a self-proclaimed expert on obesity. I know the calorie count, carb count, and protein count of most foods. I am a whiz label reader. I own two food scales.

But as you read this book you'll notice that all this knowledge has not done me much good.

So why am I writing this book at all? Because I consider myself an "obesity survivor." Despite all my failed attempts to lose and keep weight off—including gastric bypass surgery—I am not giving up. You want to know why? Because even though I'm a grandmother, and even though I'm fat, I know that deep down inside (once you work your way through all the belly rolls) there lives a hot, sexy, energetic woman who is simply not ready to settle for the fatty life. As I write this I'm fifty-five years old, and I don't expect to become any younger—but I'd prefer to enjoy my life as a woman in her fifties, not her seventies.

Right now you're probably either laughing or shaking your head, thinking, *This woman is pathetic.* Well, I'm not pathetic. I'm determined. I'm determined to live my life the way I know it was intended to be lived.

But what, you ask, what will be different this time? To begin with, honesty. In this book I will admit to the world the truths of my life, and share all my deep dark secrets. Does it make me brave to admit that I sneak-eat when no one is looking? Not really. Although I'll share things with you that most people would be mortified to have others learn, I'm not afraid of ridicule. Hell, I'm at an age where what others think about me doesn't make a whole heck of a lot of difference. Take me as is.

So: picture me standing at a pulpit in a room filled with ten thousand food sinners (perhaps one of them is you). I'm wild-eyed and passionate, with my hands stretched up to the heavens as I cry, "Confession is good for the soul!"

And that's what I'm going to do. I'm here to confess my food sins to you, loudly and succinctly. Hear me now! I am a foodie! I am at fat foodie! I promise to cleanse my soul from the demonic addiction to binge eating! Heal! Heal my soul! And for God's sake, drop some weight!

Why am I doing this? To remind you that you are not alone. Sure, there are now millions of us fatties just in the U.S. alone. But how we got here, our food eccentricities, are what shame us. And in sharing mine, I hope to help free you from yours.

Don't be afraid if you recognize yourself in these pages. We share a kinship, you and I. We understand each other. It doesn't matter what others think—besides, you'll find that they're committing the same sins as you and me. Not all the confessions in this book are mine.

Nevertheless, most of this story is about my personal journey through the world of food addiction.

It's said that if you do something that fills you with guilt, and you admit to the deed and take responsibility for it, you'll feel as if the weight of the world has been lifted from your shoulders. If that's true, then by the time we get to the end of this book I should feel very light indeed. I intend to admit how naughty I've been—justified or not—and to take full responsibility for my weight. After all, no one ever tied me up (ooh) or held me down (that's a thought) and shoved lasagna down my throat (sounds like fun...and fattening). I did all that to myself.

If you want to read more confessions like this, read on. What I say will shock some of you and amuse others—but hopefully it will give *all* of you the sense of comfort that comes from knowing you are not alone.

So grab a box of Kleenex. You might end up crying—either *for* me, or from laughing so hard *at* me. Either way, this food junkie is ready to confess.

This book was written with earnestness, honesty, and compassion. It's about the truth. It's very honest, maybe too honest, which might come back to haunt me. But what is the worst that can happen? A few people laugh at me? Fine. Other people feel embarrassed or sorry for me? That's okay, too. I hope that you, my new friends, will see yourself in me and, in doing so, recognize that you are not alone. So come one, come all. Confess your sins! Set your heart free, clear your conscience. Live like you have never lived before.

Allow me to start.

My name is Linda Misleh Wagner, and I am a true fatty....

ADMIT IT

CHAPTER 1

S he waits for her family to be seated in the family room, then makes her move. Once she's sure everyone is engrossed in the television program she creeps into the kitchen, pulls a napkin from the holder and quietly lifts the lid off the cookie jar. She wraps four chocolate-chip cookies in the napkin in such a way that the napkin looks casually bunched up.

As she passes through the family room she fakes a sneeze into the napkin, figuring that nobody would suspect her of blowing snot into a stack of cookies.

She makes her way to the bathroom, where she locks the door, puts down the lid of the toilet, sits...and devours the cookies.

Every single one of them.

Does that story sound familiar? If so, then you and I probably share the same relationship with food: we sneak behind the backs of those who care about us to indulge in an illicit relationship...but instead of meeting a paramour, our big date is with a bag of Milky Way bars. It's not just overeating, it's a clandestine love affair.

The thing is, we're not fooling anyone. As Shakira belts out in her song "Hips Don't Lie," your hips and mine clearly tell the world that we sneak-eat.

I remember sitting in my car, alone except for the enormous slice of pizza I was eating, and feeling relief that no one knew what I was doing. But I was wrong. While other people might not have known the details (until now) because they didn't actually see me scarfing down that giant wedge of pepperoni (extra cheese, of course), let's face facts: Everyone knew. People like you and me are lousy at keeping our love of food a secret. The evidence against us is as plain as day: every ounce of our excess weight is there for the world to see.

Despite this, for most of my life I've pretended that I'm part of the healthy-eating world. *Sure, I love to eat*, I tell myself, *but I'm in control of it*. Right? The only person I'm fooling is me—and I'm not even doing that very well. There's a reason I snip the labels out of my clothes, and it's not to get rid of the laundry instructions.

One day I was in my office talking to two of my coworkers about our frustrations with losing weight.

"Maybe we should stop trying so hard," I said. "Maybe we should just accept ourselves for who we are. Our weight doesn't define us as women; who we are inside is what really counts. We should be recognized and respected for all our amazing qualities, not just the shapes of our bodies."

Something along those lines.

Out loud, my coworkers half-heartedly agreed with me, but it was obvious that deep down, no matter how much they wished that size did not matter, they knew that if they were too fat they would be compared negatively with others. They would be criticized. Ostracized. They defined themselves by the width of their thighs, even if no one else did. To them, the number on the scale held position *numero uno* in the hierarchy of what mattered—and nothing could dislodge it from that spot. Their attitude seemed to be, "If you're not thin, nothing else about you matters."

How sad, I thought.

Another friend told me that if she gained five pounds she couldn't have sex with her boyfriend.

"Your boyfriend makes you feel unattractive just because you put on a few pounds?" I cried.

How horrible.

"No, not at all. In fact, he tells me he doesn't care about it; that I'm always beautiful."

"Does he mean it? Do you think he's sincere?"

"Oh, yes, he thinks I'm beautiful no matter what."

So it was my *friend* who felt too uncomfortable and embarrassed to have sex unless she looked a certain way. Her opinion of herself was destroying her self-worth...and perhaps even her relationship.

How tragic.

And it is. It's tragic that so many of us are hung up on physical appearances and let our size determine our self-worth. It's tragic that we're scared we'll be judged by our weight instead of who we are as human beings.

And you know what? We *are* judged by our weight. Tragic or not, sad or not, we're all judged by our size, at least at first. Even by ourselves. We might as well admit it.

It's difficult for binge eaters like you and me to really face what we're doing to ourselves, which is why I'm doing it now. By baring my own soul and being completely honest, perhaps I can accept my binge eating as just another a problem to solve rather than the definition of who I am. And perhaps if you see a bit of your experience in mine, you can, too.

This is how we get out of our fat suits: layer by layer. We will start with the "jacket" and work our way down. You know the jacket I'm talking about: it hangs on us, all loose and flabby. Although it has no real shape it tries to be sexy and seductive. But who are we kidding? We're not referring to five extra pounds here. Do we really believe that thighs that develop a rash from rubbing together are sexy? Does anyone truly think that the muffin-top rolls around our middles make the objects of our desire lick their lips in anticipation? Come on!

I'm not going fight the truth any longer. I'm exhausted from pretending that I'm exactly the person I want to be. I'm tired of pretending to have a good relationship with food. I don't. It's time to come out of the baked goods cabinet and confess to the world that I have a real addiction. As hard as I try to fight temptation and ignore the irrational cravings I know will do me harm, there are times when I just can't seem to get past the desire to eat. On those occasions my willpower takes a coffee break (I don't even like coffee) and I can hear the evil cookies in the cupboards or the leftover spaghetti in the fridge calling, "Eat me.... Devour me...."

So let's break the shackles of denial that weigh us down and run free. (Well, I'll *imagine* running free. I don't actually run, ever. Walk fast, but never run.) At least metaphorically, let's stop hiding behind layers of...well, layers.

No, let me say it clearly: *fat.* Layers of fat. Lots and lots of fat. We hate it and wish desperately to rid ourselves of it. We fight to lose weight—and sometimes we succeed, only to regain it not just once but over and over again: losing and gaining, losing and gaining.

We all love to eat, and many of us also share my *addiction* to food. Perhaps you even have food rituals. For instance, every Monday night might be pizza night for you (for me, personally, any moment of the day is pizza night). Or you might have stashes of food concealed around the house. (Ever hide a candy bar between folded panties in your lingerie drawer? Come on; I know I'm not the only one out there....)

These are only some of the reasons that the battle to lose weight is rarely won by anyone for long. As much as we abhor the fat suits that encase the svelte physiques of our dreams, we go on wearing them like an old pair of comfortable jeans, soft, loose and familiar. In these suits we feel safe. But we must ask ourselves: Why does keeping our fat suits on make us feel safe? And safe from what?

Do those baggy jeans hide our secrets, our desires, our deep needs? Do they give us wisdom in rough times? Do they protect us from ourselves when we're at our worst? Do they make our problems go away? Nope, not one bit—and you and I both know it. If each ounce of excess fat on my body could somehow solve one world problem, trust me, global warming would cease, Israelis and Palestinians would join hands and sing "Kumbaya," and North Korea would throw its gates open to all visitors. No: the reason we keep wearing those fat jeans is that nothing else in our closet fits us without popping a button or cutting off our circulation.

Look, we know we're fat. But we also believe that we, like non-fatties, should be able to enjoy eating without worry or guilt. Sorry. That's like saying an alcoholic can enjoy a single social drink along with everyone else. We need to acknowledge our dysfunctional relationship with food, and then decide whether or not we accept our weight. If not, then what are we going to do to change the number on the scale? We should be able to make better choices with every meal, every snack, and still indulge occasionally in the sinful yummies the world has to offer. Eat what we want, but be in control. *Genuinely* in control.

That's what we should be able to do. But we don't.

Which is why it's time to think of ourselves not as obese people but as obesity survivors.

What is an obesity survivor? Someone who has dealt with obesity for most of his or her life; tried almost every diet known to mankind; perhaps gone so far as to have surgery to fix the eating problem. Above all, an obesity survivor is someone who refuses to give up, no matter what.

For me, fighting the battle of obesity has been lifelong drudgery—and it's a war I intend to win. They say that half the battle is admitting you have a problem. Perhaps if we get to the root of why we obsess over food, we will take away the power food has over us and will instead empower ourselves to take charge of our own lives. Why let food have power over us when *we* should have power over *food*?

When she eats out with friends, she often suggests they go to an all-you-can-eat buffet. "Buffets have something to please everyone," she says. It's true. She knows it's true because on more than one occasion she's eaten there by herself—during off hours so nobody she knows will spot her stuffing thousands of calories into her already bloated body.

"Also," she adds, "buffets are great for people trying to watch what they eat." This is a good selling point because not only she, but all of her friends, are on diets. They always seem to be on diets. "We can have as much salad and meat as we want to and just stay away from the carbs."

Well, maybe she'll have just a little pasta salad and a small taste of cake....

TOMATOES AND THIN MINTS

CHAPTER 2

He hands his newborn daughter carefully to his mother-in-law, who looks upon her first granddaughter with joy. The baby weighs only five pounds, fourteen ounces. She has huge, dark, almond-shaped eyes, little bow lips, and lots of thick, wavy black hair. Her features hold the promise that she will someday grow into a beautiful woman.

To her parents and grandmother she is the most gorgeous baby ever born. They could not imagine that this tiny infant of less than six pounds will come to suffer from weight control issues for most of her life.

I was born in Washington, D.C. on May 30th, 1958, on the way to a picnic. My mother, father, and an assortment of uncles and cousins were crammed into a car, heading out of town for a Memorial Day celebration, when I decided to make my debut.

My dad, who had emigrated to the U.S. from Palestine after World War II, turned the car around fast and sped back toward Doctors Hospital in Washington. Not even born, and already I had a posse! I'm told that no one complained about missing the picnic.

Most Palestinian families want their firstborn child to be a son, firstly so he can carry on the family name, and secondly because in Palestinian culture, boys simply have more implied value than girls.

But it wasn't like that for my dad. Nobody doubted his elation when he announced that he had a daughter.

Not surprisingly, he liked to call me "Princess."

My mom, on the other hand, kept me grounded. Born in Vermont in 1936 to a Palestinian father and a Syrian mother, she'd been raised in New Haven, Connecticut. Before meeting my dad at a mutual cousin's wedding, she'd worked in a bridal boutique. Because of her tiny, perfect figure and exotic looks, the boutique's owners had used her as a model for their gowns whenever a regular model didn't show up at a fashion show.

My dad was a debonair man, short, chubby and very handsome. When he came to America from Ramallah, Palestine, he brought with him his old world values and devotion, and he commanded and earned respect everywhere he went. He was astute at business and successful in all his endeavors.

Once married, my parents moved to Arlington, Virginia, where my dad and his brother Ned opened several businesses. Meanwhile my mother worked as a secretary for both Senator John F. Kennedy and General McNamara, and quit only after I came along.

My father had brought my grandfather to America with him, and eventually my grandmother and my dad's brothers joined the immigrants. Dad's sisters married and they, too, eventually settled in the United States.

My Ramallah ancestry can be traced to the founding of the city almost eighteen hundred years ago. According to legend, one of my ancestors refused to marry his best friend's daughter because the girls' family was Muslim and my ancestor was Christian. Although my ancestor meant no insult, his Christian beliefs were strong, and Islam was a relatively new religion at the time.

But the result was catastrophic: a battle ensued, friend against friend, and ultimately my ancestor's friend, a Muslim sheik, sent a battalion of mounted men to find and kill my ancestor and all his kin.

But my ancestor discovered that the soldiers were coming and set a trap. He and his family and supporters made their way across the Jordan River, leaving behind an array of sharpened spikes sunk into the riverbed just beneath the water. With a thunderous roar the enemy force galloped full speed into the river.

Spikes tore into horseflesh and the Muslims were thrown into the river, which turned red with the blood of man and beast.

My ancestor and his clan escaped to the west and settled a piece of land ten miles north of Jerusalem, thus founding the town of Ramallah. My ancestor soon met and married a beautiful Christian girl who bore him five sons. Ramallah is now a bustling city housing people of many faiths and devotions, including Christians, Muslims and Jews, yet many people of the city trace their bloodlines back to one or another of my ancestor's sons.

This story brings us to a crucial issue: the way I was raised. Throughout its long history my family was always hard-working and industrious. My father and his relatives came to the United States to join in the success of the American lifestyle. They embraced this country, where the opportunities for people willing to work hard were endless. After beginning with a carpet-cleaning business and a restaurant, my father and his brothers went into the grocery trade. By the time my father retired he was the landlord of many properties that he and his brothers had developed in San Diego, California.

My own childhood was spent in the grocery business. In 1963 we moved from Washington to San Francisco, where we owned a store on the corner of Haight and Ashbury—the iconic intersection at the center of the hippie universe. I remember my mother bringing my sister and brothers and me down to visit my dad at the store, outside of which hippies were hanging around passing out flowers.

My father and uncle worked from six a.m. to midnight, seven days a week, until they got some help in the store; then one would work the first shift from six a.m. to six p.m., and the other would work from noon until midnight. Best of all, they could finally take every other Sunday off!

On those Sundays, after church we'd go visit relatives, most of whom also owned grocery stores. My aunts and uncles were very kind to us kids; they'd hand us brown paper bags and turned us loose in the candy aisles of their stores. Although my mother would admonish us to only take one candy bar each, my aunt would shush her and insist that we fill our bags.

So, while my mother and father sat on milk crates drinking Arabic coffee from tiny porcelain demitasse cups, my siblings and I would run around the store, playing hide and seek. It wasn't until my mother and father insisted that we settle down and sit like ladies and gentlemen that we would begin to devour our candy bars.

After our parents finished their coffee, we would all leave and go to the next relative's grocery store, where the process would be repeated.

Given how hard everyone worked, this was the only way our extended family could socialize. By the time we got home and Mom heated dinner, we kids would be hungry despite all the candy and Cracker Jacks we had consumed. How could we not be, with the aromas of exotic spices wafting throughout the house? Most meals were a combination of lamb, rice, salt, pepper, and allspice. Sauces made with yogurt, garlic, and mint. There were tomatoes, and oh, the aroma of homemade Arabic bread. So delicious!

The rage over pita bread today was unheard of when I was a kid. My friends at school would look at my sandwich made up of pita and whatever was stuffed inside it, and think my lunch very strange...until they came over and tried my mom's cooking. After that they wanted to eat at my house all the time.

Food is a significant part of all cultures, but for Arabs, meals lie at the center of every event. Men and women both are excellent cooks; for a woman it is a sign of shame to not cook well.

When I was a child my personal love of food was not a problem. Despite my diminutive size at birth I developed early. I was solidly built but not fat. Genetics accounts for much of this. Arab kids are not like European kids; Arab kids are usually thicker in build and generally go through puberty at a much younger age. Kids of European descent tend to be light, gangly, skinny. At the age of nine I, on the other hand, was wearing a child's size fourteen while my friends were wearing ten and twelve at most. Still, I never saw myself as fat, and no one ever called me fatso or fatty.

In November of 1968 we moved to San Diego because my dad and uncle felt that in San Francisco "the times, they were a-changin'" too much and too fast. The hippie culture with its drug use and free love was taking over the Haight-Ashbury district, and my father was concerned about the influence it would have on his kids. He believed that San Diego offered a more conservative, wholesome environment.

We settled in University City, a San Diego community where many of our cousins already lived. Nowadays over one hundred families of my first, second, and third cousins live in University City, and we're all very close-knit.

Living in such a large extended family was fun; I grew up always feeling loved and supported. The situation created many occasions for us to gather...and eat. Never mind holidays; there were endless weddings, bridal showers, baby showers, christenings, birthdays, funerals.

And they all involved food.

Tata Nazha clears a space on the enormous table to make room for another platter. The table is already heavily laden with sliced leg of lamb, stuffed grape leaves, stuffed squash, and kibbeh—*lamb ground up with onions and spices and patted down in a deep pan. Next, sautéed lamb chunks and chopped onions with salt, pepper, and allspice with browned pine nuts are mixed and placed on the bottom layer of patties, followed by a top layer of the ground meat-and-onion mixture. Finally, melted rendered butter is drizzled over the top layer, and the* kibbeh *is baked until browned.*

Other staples on the table include homemade hummus and olives—usually picked off neighbors' trees—cheeses, nuts, fruits and sambousek *(Arab* empanadas*). And of course there are also meat pies, spinach pies and a salad called* taboullah*, all accompanied by homemade Arabic bread, and we ain't talkin' store bought Pita, baby.*

Room on the table has to be made for dessert, which will of course include Aunt Mary's famous kannafeh*, made of crushed shredded wheat mixed with rendered butter. Half the shredded wheat will go on the bottom of a large round cake pan, followed by a layer of a cheese with a ricotta-like consistency, and topped by more of the shredded wheat. This will be baked until golden, and then drenched in a homemade syrup consisting of two parts sugar to one part water and a tablespoon of lemon juice, all boiled for seven minutes.*

Tata Nazha places a tray of baklava *and another of Arabic sugar cookies (*garibeh*) on the table. She takes a good look to make sure nothing is missing, then walks to the family room and informs my father that everything is ready so he may announce that dinner is served.*

This was typical of the dinners served during special occasions in my family.

Sounds like a great deal of food, doesn't it? Our cultural philosophy is that we would rather have too much than too little, and it's always better to be prepared with extra just in case someone unexpectedly stops by. Anything not eaten at the time will serve as leftovers, giving the women a much-needed day off from cooking—Arabic food is very time-consuming to make.

I remember the night when everyone—over twenty-five of us—was invited to my Uncle Ned's house, which was located right next door to ours, for homemade pizza. Ned had built a stone oven into the hillside in his backyard. All day long he prepared Arabic bread while two large pots of freshly-made tomato sauce simmered on the stovetop. My aunt had pepperoni, sausage and fresh vegetables cut up and ready to top the pizzas.

An assembly line formed. One person rolled out the dough, the next spread the sauce, and the next topped the pizza with cheese, followed by another adding an assortment of vegetables and meats. My Uncle Ed and Uncle Sam then carried the pizzas out to the back yard, where Uncle Ned was waiting to bake them.

The result was so fresh and delicious that long after reaching the point where you'd eaten so much you thought you might actually explode, you just had to take one more slice. No one could resist the melted mozzarella dripping off the sides of a slice of pizza built on homemade Arabic bread.

My mother's brother, Richard, was visiting from Connecticut that day. As I sat in the family room trying to quietly digest all the pizza I had eaten, Uncle Richard staggered in through the patio door. He looked to be in agony as he lowered himself to the floor.

"Are you alright, Uncle Richard?" I asked.

He moaned. "I can't move. I can barely breathe."

"What's wrong?" Now I was really scared.

"I ate too much. I ate too much pizza. I can't move...."

Uncle Richard fell into a pizza-induced sleep right there on the floor.

The rest of us found our own corners of the room and pretty much stayed put until bedtime. If pain can be good, that was the best kind. I was fifteen or sixteen years old at the time, and still remember that evening with fondness. Great food served up by a great family.

Terrific memories...but as you can see, food was the reason to get everyone together. And we didn't need a wedding or a holiday to gather. All it took was for someone to say, "Come over; we're cooking something you'll love."

If you believe all this contributed to my weight problems, you could be right...but I actually don't think so. In fact I only mention it because although many of the people in my family love to eat, many of them manage to keep their weight at a respectable level. My sister, both brothers and mom all managed to stay at reasonable weights for many years; not until they were older did they have to battle to keep their weights down.

So what's my excuse? What drove me to out-of-control eating behavior? Things were good with my family. I had great friends. I certainly don't remember any single event that might have been a catalyst for future binge eating, apart from the fact that my weight problems began at the same time I began going through puberty—at about age eleven.

To add to the mystery, I had always been active. I played girls' softball and took modern dance classes. I loved to ride my bike; cruising for miles with the wind blowing through my hair felt like freedom to me. In other words, I was no couch potato.

I also helped my dad on weekends and during the summer in our family's grocery store. For me it was fun. I loved getting to know the customers, some of whom became like family to us. The same was true of employees. We employed a full-time butcher who my brother, Anton, teased unmercifully. Anton would sneak into the milk box and, using his slingshot, send an empty pistachio shell flying across the meat department right into the backside of the butcher.

The best—and, in retrospect, probably the worst—part of working in the store was the access to free candy and baked goods. The store sold penny red and black licorice from a shelf behind the counter next to the Bazooka bubblegum and Thin Mints. I used to take two Red Vines and one Black vine, braid them together, and eat the resulting rope.

I can't tell you how many boxes of Bazooka I went through. And the Thin Mints? They somehow disappeared every time I took over the cash register. It got to the point that my Uncle Ned had to tell my brother, my cousins, and me to stop eating all the profits.

In addition to the candy, the Hostess and Dolly Madison baked goods cast their seductive spell over me. Here's a confession: When I took a break from work I'd grab a magazine, hold it at an angle against my chest, and walk casually past the Zingers. Along the way I'd grab a package and pin it between my chest and the magazine while I strolled to the back room. There I'd eagerly devour those processed, Satan-Sugared Sweet Cakes (my personal name for Zingers).

One of my favorite parts about working at our family business was lunchtime with my dad. I'd make tuna fish sandwiches, which we'd eat at a homemade wooden table while sitting on milk crates. My dad would share stories of his life with me; I especially loved to hear about his childhood.

He also gave me advice. "Linda, always strive for the very best for yourself. Want it for the guy next to you just as much. This way you are both happy and doing well."

He lived this motto, as I do. But reaching for perfection all the time has a price. The house must be spotless. Every single meal must be special. As a woman, I must take care of other people's needs and wants before my own in order to feel I'm making a difference in their lives. If I cook a nice meal, set a nice table and make sure everyone is comfortable, I'm showing love and respect for both others and myself. I'm also creating an environment worthy of coming home to. One's home is a sanctuary; a family should always return to a welcoming and comforting environment.

I also had my mother's example to live up to. She would always tuck her children in at night and listen to our problems, even when she was bone tired herself. Her family's needs always came before her own.

From the beginning I, too, was raised to be a good wife and mother. Even though my parents encouraged education (they expected all of us to be college graduates), for my sister and me the most noble career we could choose was that of wife and mother—outstanding wives and mothers, of course.

My father also taught me to be a leader and not a follower. This lesson, along with the underlying threat that he might kill me (not literally), kept me from giving in to peer pressure. No drugs, no smoking, no alcohol...and above all no fraternizing with boys.

She hands her father the tomatoes as he loads the produce display. She can tell he knows something's on her mind, but is waiting for her to find a way to ask him.

"Daddy?" she finally says.

"Yes, sweetheart?"

"Daddy, why won't you let me date? There's a real nice boy at school that I like a lot, and he asked me to the school dance. Dad, he's real nice, and he would never do anything inappropriate. Please say yes, Daddy."

Without hesitation he picks up a ripe tomato. "Linda, you see this tomato? Do you see how beautiful and perfect it is?"

"Yes." She tries not to sound impatient. What does a tomato have to do with her?

"Today, customers will come in to buy tomatoes. They will pick them up, and they will pinch the tomato and squeeze the tomato and pinch some more. Do you know what you have then at the end of the day?"

"What, Dad?"

"Bruised tomatoes." He gazes into her eyes. "I don't want you to become a bruised tomato."

Tell me how to argue with logic like that. It is impossible.

If you don't think I was frustrated by this kind of thing, think again. Consider the time my parents and I went to a big Arab-American party. Such parties were formal affairs, usually held in the ballroom of a nice hotel. These events were catered, and featured Arabic singers and musicians as well as a DJ playing American music.

Despite the formality they were a lot of fun, especially since they were one of the few occasions on which a "nice Arab girl" like me would be allowed to talk to and dance with boys; after all, we were being chaperoned by twelve hundred people.

On this particular occasion I was sitting at a table with my friends when I looked up and saw my dad glaring at me from his seat clear across the ballroom. I pulled my cocktail dress tight across my lap and tucked it under my thighs, but when I looked up again, my father's expression hadn't changed. I sat even straighter and made sure that not too much cleavage was showing (we were not allowed to show too much cleavage, or bare backs, or stomachs, or thighs), but still he glared.

Finally I couldn't take it any longer. I got up and walked to him across the room. To my surprise, he smiled.

"What's wrong?" I said.

"What do you mean?"

"You've been glaring at me. Nothing was showing, and I was sitting like a lady. Why are you glaring at me?"

"*Habiti* ("sweetheart"), I wasn't looking at you. I was looking at something across the room behind you."

"Oh...."

If you need help understanding the picture I'm trying to paint for you, I'll be very clear. Guilt! I was raised by two wonderful people who were also strict disciplinarians; they instilled enough guilt in their children for us to think twice about messing up our lives.

If I make it sound like they abused me, they did not. They didn't have to. For me, the idea of letting my folks down was worse punishment than anything they could actually do to me. They kept me in line with nothing more than a look (a skill my own children would tell you I inherited).

If you were to ask my parents about the way they'd managed my early life, they would tell you I was being silly; they only did what any parent does to teach their children right from wrong. *Oy!* Jewish and Italian mothers had nothing on my parents when it came to laying on the guilt.

By now I'm sure you're wondering how any of this translates to my turning to food. What drove me to self-medicating with my drug of choice? I could tease you and say it was because I wasn't allowed to indulge in drugs or alcohol, or to smoke cigarettes—which I wasn't. But the truth is, there were several factors involved.

First, expectations. I was brought up knowing that I had to meet a long string of expectations, including being conscientious and considerate, getting good grades, learning to cook and clean so I'd make a good wife, and getting an education.

Second: judgment. I felt that if I did not excel at whatever I did, I'd be negatively judged by my parents and other authority figures in my life. Since I never wanted to disappoint my parents, my teachers, my friends, or for that matter anyone else, I strove always to be the best at anything I tried.

Third: guilt. I've already touched on this, but guilt can take many forms. Such as: nice Palestinian girls keep away from boys. That's just how it is; we're expected to guard our virtue until we're married. One's reputation as a "nice Palestinian girl" could be destroyed by simply *talking* to a boy for too long. It worked like this: If someone from a "good family" saw a girl talking too long to a boy or being too flirty, that could prevent anyone from the "good family" ever asking for the girl's hand in marriage.

Not that I, personally, had many opportunities to ruin my reputation, even if I wanted to. With a family the size of mine, there were eyes everywhere.

I could never go out without running into a relative. Usually several relatives.

As a result I grew up under constant, loving pressure to be a good girl and good student, to prepare to be a good wife and mother, and to ignore the impulses of my free spirit that wanted to date and kiss boys and experience the world. At one point my parents were genuinely afraid I'd run off to Hollywood to become an actress and shame my family (because as everyone knows, in order to be a movie star a woman has to get naked on screen sooner or later). My parents no doubt found this particular fear legitimate because I'd been writing plays and acting them out since I was a very small child, and in school I took four years of drama.

Here's the irony: because my parents were so strict, I never even *considered* rebelling. The cost was just too high. As a result, I never felt like the typical American teenager. For example, when I asked to have a boy/girl party for my sixteenth birthday, my dad suggested an alternative: a trip to Las Vegas with six of my girlfriends.

"I will take you," he said. "We will stay at Caesar's Palace, and I will take you and your friends to the Bacchanal Room for dinner. You can hang out at the pool and shop every day. My treat."

"Dad, why can't I have a regular party with boys and girls?"

"*No boys!*"

So... no boys. Instead, they threw me a surprise party and invited all of my closest girlfriends. When my parents said no, they meant no. Disobeying them was unthinkable; it would be letting them down.

The part of me that dreads disappointing anyone I love has been prevalent throughout my life. This overwhelming conscientiousness is an integral part of my personality—and stems from the messages I received throughout my childhood.

What about you? Take a look at the messages your parents fed you while you were growing up. Think about the influence that teachers and others you looked up to had upon you. Then think about how you distilled those messages. You might discover that the way you live now is a reflection of these inner messages.

Add to that the pressure of a skill most of us have also mastered: being too hard on ourselves. This is especially common amongst overeaters. Different people react in different ways to the same stimuli. As a young person I felt intense pressure to live up to other peoples' expectations of me before I ever defined my expectations for myself. My parents did not drive me to overindulge in food; my own insecurities pushed me in that direction.

When you're brought up to stifle your inner rebel, you don't make too many mistakes...at least, not at the time. Frankly, I was a great kid—although I'm sure my mom would insist that I was also the hardest to raise because I was so free-spirited, always gallivant-ing around and never sitting still.

She's right. I did want to gallivant, and to this day I hate sitting still. But striving always to be the good child, stifling your ambitions, and constantly wor-rying about letting others down only teaches you to let *yourself* down. My spiral into the world of obesity began because I never learned to fight for myself. Where was the fireball inside me willing to set bound-aries for others, stand up for myself, and *fight back*?

Don't get me wrong. I know that my parents were trying to protect me and educate me to carry on our family values and traditions. I love and respect that. The problem is that I was born into two cultures: one a little too strict for my liking, the other too perverse (hello, I grew up in the sixties and seventies; free love and drugs!). I never really fit into either.

But that was long ago, and at some point we all need to temper the messages from our childhoods with the common sense and experience of adulthood—taking care to also apply a sense of understanding, not blame. The problem is that by the time we finally begin to understand these concepts, most of us have already established deeply entrenched habits to fill childhood voids and frustrations.

Habits like overeating.

Only as we mature does wisdom (some, at least!) come to us. Where was it in our teens? If only back then we were capable of grasping pearls of wisdom as they floated past, there would be a lot fewer people suffering as adults from addiction and self-abuse. We would feel less insecure, appreciate ourselves more for who we are, and have a stronger sense of self-confidence. Kids would take more responsibility for their own actions and blame others less (how novel would that be?). And above all, we would accept the consequences of our actions.

But no matter what childhood messages we were raised with, no matter how difficult our early years, sooner or later we have to decide what kind of lives we want to live from now on. We must learn to channel what works for us and discard what does not, without turning to addictive coping patterns.

In one breath my parents would make me feel very loved, but in the next my dad could make me feel that there were strings attached to his love. At times that made me angry—and then I would feel guilty for the anger. Of course, I know Dad was doing his best—and, in fact, most of the messages he drove home made me into a good and wonderful person (I'm stating facts, not bragging). But other messages created a pattern within me of never taking care of myself first. Never putting my own feelings—which, after all, should be most important to me—at the top of my list.

But the human mind has a way of making its needs known.

No one else is home. She has the house all to herself. She rummages through the freezer to see if there's any ice cream. Crap! Someone finished it off!

She opens the refrigerator. Fruit, fruit, fruit! Nothing but fruit. She wants something REALLY sweet. There must be cookies somewhere. After all, her family owns a grocery store and brings home boxes of food every night.

Nope, no cookies. Well, then, she'll have to improvise. She takes a baby food bowl out of the cabinet and spoons in powdered sugar. Then she grabs a bottle of Aunt Jemima's Maple Syrup and squirts a huge dollop into the bowl. She mixes it into the powdered sugar, scoops out a spoonful and swallows it.

Hmmmmm...it might not be exceptionally delicious, but it certainly is sweet.

It will do for now.

DON'T LET THEM EAT CAKE

CHAPTER 3

She stands in line in the school cafeteria, a dime ready in her hand. Ever since she discovered that they sell Frosties in the cafeteria, she makes sure she has ten cents in her pocket every day.

Her parents have expressed concern about her weight. Although she's only eleven going on twelve, over the past year she's put on close to twenty pounds. Her parents don't think she's interested in making changes to her diet.

They've tried to talk to her about it, but she always reacts as if they're nagging her. If anything, when they speak she eats even more.

She just can't seem to stop herself.

That was me standing in that cafeteria line every day, Monday through Friday. I was at an awkward age for a young pubescent girl growing up in a strict Middle Eastern family.

My father didn't want me to get too close to Americans; he was afraid they would influence me too much. Especially, of course, boys. He didn't trust boys at all. He knew I had a bit of a wild, flirty side, so he felt he had to keep tight reins on me—to protect me, naturally.

I was never allowed to have sleepovers at my place or spend the night at a friend's house. My father always asked if the friend had brothers. If they did, the answer was an automatic "No." He didn't trust fathers much either. I didn't understand why he was so concerned. It wasn't until I was much older, married, and had my own children that I realized what troubled him so much—especially after I watched a few *Dateline* shows about men you would never suspect of being child molesters. Now all I can say is, "Thank you, *Baba* (Dad)."

But at the time, my parents' protectiveness made me feel constricted and suppressed. I wanted to take drama classes and dance classes—and did so, although as I've said, my passion for the performing arts troubled my parents. Dad, of course, didn't like the way the boys in drama behaved, always chasing the girls around and grabbing at us (lucky us). In addition, my parents felt that my head already floated too far in the clouds, that I was living in a fantasy world. And maybe I was—but I loved the creativity that flowed through me when I did performing arts.

The arts were where I wanted to make my living—although I never did plan to run off to Hollywood, as my parents feared. Instead I imagined owning a clothing boutique where I would sell my own designs to well-dressed rich women. The boutique would be located in the high-end coastal enclave of La Jolla, specifically on Prospect Street. Women would come in and sit in a sunken living room, sipping mimosas and eating their choice of white- or milk chocolate-covered strawberries while models walked the runway showing off my designs. The adjacent playroom would be fully staffed so moms could shop undisturbed. My clients would choose an outfit they wanted and be fitted for it, after which a professional makeup artist would assist them in choosing the right cosmetics to complement their complexions and the outfit they had selected. Of course there would also be a perfume counter, hairdresser, manicurist. This would be a full-service boutique.

Oh, the dreams we have within.

But my fantasy of the boutique was never taken seriously by my parents, and over time it faded in contrast to my other, very well-supported ambition: to marry a nice guy from the Ramallah community and have a big family. In my dreams I had even seen the man I would wed, standing at the foot of a long, elegant staircase staring up at me as I swept down the steps in a chic evening gown. You could say I was a sensitive kid trying to bridge two worlds. I wanted the best of both, and blamed myself when I came up short in either.

On the other hand, how did I expect anyone else to take me seriously when I was not taking care of myself? By eighth grade I had doubled the twenty pounds I'd gained between sixth and seventh grades, and by the end of ninth grade my weight was up to 195 pounds.

How did this happen? As I said, I was an active kid. Apart from riding my bike, playing softball, and dancing on the school dance team, I played racquetball like a fiend. On the other hand, for each of these activities except for dance team (who wants to see a fat dancer?), food was part of the reward. It's ironic: we work out and develop a good, dripping sweat, only to go to the nearest restaurant, ice cream parlor, or drugstore to reward ourselves for all our hard work.

Then there was the environmental issue. The joke around my house was that during our huge family get-togethers with all that delicious food, the main topic of conversation was the need to lose weight. Yet I never saw anyone in my family take a walk after dinner to burn off the calories they had just consumed.

Eventually one of my uncles went on a verbal rampage about it, declaring that everyone in the family was too fat. He said we should stop having birthday cakes; none of us needed to eat cake. I asked him if he really thought we'd all gotten fat off a piece of cake. He thought I was being a smartass, but I was serious.

Let me embrace the truth: I come from a whole family of eaters. Although we've all owned gym memberships at one point or another, we're a fat clan. In fact, I used to refer to the Family Fitness chain of gyms as "Family Fatness." At the time I thought it was funny.

But not when I was fourteen. Fourteen years old and weighing almost two hundred pounds? The extra weight served only to make me run slower in gym class (and I already hated to run). Despite my dreams of someday owning a trendy clothing boutique, I had to shop in the Women's section of the department store. To make matters worse, the styles available for fat girls, especially young fat girls, were awful and embarrassing: tops made from ugly fabrics and elastic-waist stretch pants sewn from the worst of polyester. I wanted to dress young and hip, like Marcia Brady of the *Brady Bunch*. Instead I looked like Alice, the housekeeper. It sucked to be fourteen and fat.

But I didn't do anything about it until I overheard the boy I had a crush on call me a "fat ass." (Jeff Cudmore, wherever you are, you tore my heart to pieces.)

That insult made me actually take action. I was sick and tired of being a fat teenager. For the first time, I hated my body more than I loved to eat. No matter what delectable food was on the table, and no matter what the occasion—birthdays, weddings, family bar-beques—nothing, *nothing!* would stop me from losing weight this time.

On April 23 of her ninth grade year she joins Weight Watchers—and over the course of the next summer loses over fifty pounds.

KILLER CURVES

CHAPTER 4

*O*n her first day of school as a tenth grader she wears gray pants and a gray, white, and burgundy checkered blouse that cinches tightly around her new, tiny waist. Tom Locke and the rest of the athletes from the football team take one look at her and don't even try to keep their appreciation of her new figure off their faces. Desire gleams in their eyes.

Heady! That's how it feels. Very heady!

I'll tell you this: when I started tenth grade I had curves I was proud of. In retrospect, the process sounds so easy. **The more weight I lost, the more I moved. The more I moved, the more weight I lost, and the slimmer and harder my body became.** Don't tell my father, but I loved walking around in leotards when coming to or leaving dance class. For the first time in my life I felt foxy (the term used back then to describe a really hot chick). Foxy, empowered, sexy.

As a bonus, I also loved the respect and pride I felt coming from my parents and other family members.

So high school that year was great. Despite my parents' apprehensions, I got heavily involved in both drama and dance. I was popular, even though I was not allowed to do anything with the popular kids. Best of all, one of my middle school friends, Sandra Ducheny, became my best friend. Sandra is of Puerto Rican descent and had a strict upbringing not unlike my own. Neither of us was allowed to date or go to friends' parties, so we understood each other. We both managed to have fun with other kids...flirting... teasing...and then went home to be the good little girls our parents expected us to be.

Both of us also went from being fatties in middle school to not-so-fatties in high school. The rewards were wonderful, but make no mistake: losing all that weight and keeping it off required sacrifice. Here's what I ate every day: for breakfast, a slice of buttered sourdough toast and a piece of fruit; for lunch, a golden delicious apple and a Tab (the first Diet Coke); and for dinner whatever my mother made—but I ate my portion in a bowl left over from when I was a baby; literally a baby food bowl.

The sacrifice seemed well worth it. The attention I was getting from men made me feel incredibly womanly, although there were times it was frightening as well.

That first year after I lost weight my father took me to San Francisco for the annual Ramallah convention. It was a huge gathering of more than five thousand people. I was fifteen and feeling fabulous and powerful.

The convention was held at the Hyatt Regency at Fisherman's Wharf. One night I spent the evening dancing with several Ramallah guys. One young man in particular, much older than me—about 27 years old—asked me to dance. I will say only his first name, Mike. We danced to "Smoke On The Water."

After the dance, one of my close cousins, Jamal, warned me to stay away from Mike. He said Mike was known for drinking too much, womanizing, and even drug use. I appreciated the warning and spent the rest of the evening avoiding Mike, who had taken quite a liking to me.

At two a.m., while my girl cousins from New York and I were sitting on the third floor sitting area talking, a very drunken Mike came up to me and said he wanted to marry me. Right then. "We'll go to Tahoe or Reno and get married right away. Come on; I have a van waiting outside."

I told him "no," but he refused to take that as an answer.

He grabbed me and began to literally drag me, in my evening gown, toward the escalators. My cousins from New York and many other people started yelling at him to release me. He refused.

Suddenly my father and several of my uncles appeared. My father grabbed Mike and pulled him off me. I had never seen my father so angry. He picked Mike up by the front of his tuxedo and lifted him over the balustrade, ready to drop Mike the three stories to the ground.

It was my uncles who talked my father out of dropping Mike. Instead, they pulled drunken Mike back onto his feet and my father punched him in the face. Again it was my uncles who pulled my dad off of Mike.

Some of Mike's uncles came over and escorted their nephew out of sight. Where he went after that I don't know, nor do I care. I certainly didn't see him over the remaining days of the convention.

My father made sure I was okay, and we all decided it was time to get casual. Everyone went upstairs to their rooms to change into tee shirts and jeans. We were all to meet afterwards down in the lobby to talk.

My 13 year-old cousin Abe from New York was worried about me after what had happened, and offered to come up with me and wait while I changed. He was like a brother to me, so I didn't think much of it.

In my hotel room, I was grabbing jeans and a tee shirt and heading for the bathroom to change when my father knocked on the door and stuck his head into the room to make sure I was okay. The room was dark except for the light in the dressing area and bathroom, so what he saw was a mannish silhouette sitting on the edge of my bed.

My father leaped on Abe and was about to strike him when I shouted, "Dad! What are you doing? What's wrong?"

He scowled. "What is Abe doing in your room?"

"He wanted to make sure I was safe; he was waiting for me to change clothes in the bathroom."

I thought my father was going to have a heart attack. "Abe, please wait in the hallway."

Abe stepped outside, shaking, his lower lip quivering.

My dad turned to me. "Sit down."

Boy oh boy, did I get an earful, gently but firmly, as my father explained why a nice girl does not allow a man into her hotel room for any reason.

All I could say was, "Abe's not a man. He's a boy."

My father was both worried and exasperated with me. I learned a monumental lesson then about how men think and dads react when it comes to protecting the virtue and reputations of their daughters.

I learned another lesson as well: all this attention because I'd lost weight and developed a hot figure? Sheesh! Holy shmoly!

If you think this incident made me turn back to food and put my protective fat suit back on, think again. All it did was serve to make me want to stay thin. Back to hardly eating for me.

The Weight Watchers program was very structured, but it worked. I kept the weight off throughout high school and the first two years of college—almost six years. Despite the difficulty in doing it, and even though my parents would not allow me to date or appear amongst the Arab community as anything but a nice virginal girl, I cannot say I was unhappy. I felt so great in my body that all the restrictions on the rest of my life did not seem overbearing. After all, a constrained life was normal for me. The way I was raised was no different than all my Arab girlfriends, not to mention my best friend Sandie.

And I *did* want to marry a nice Arab man. Although my American guy friends were good-looking, they were far more immature than Arab high school boys. Arabs raise their kids to mature and take responsibility at a very young age. Also, expectations in the Arab community are very clear-cut: get a good education, marry a nice Arab and have a nice Arab family. This business (as my father would say) of "gallivanting," traveling around after high school, and drinking too much at college parties was a waste of time.

According to my father, all the things I felt l was missing out on in life—romance, parties, nightclubbing—would become available to me after I married. My husband and I would develop a real love built on respect and mutual goals. "The love American-born women talk about," my father said, "where they leap from boyfriend to boyfriend—that's not real love." To him, even the experience of "falling in love" was not love; it was just lust. He insisted that the love I told him I felt, love for some of the guys I knew, Arab or American, was based on physical attraction and nothing more. "Real love comes from struggling together to build a mutual life and raise a family."

Although I didn't buy into everything my father said, I did trust and believe in him. After all, every day I saw the results of his devotion to our family. So I felt I had no option but to do as he asked.

The reason I bring up this way of thinking is that it steered my life in various ways, both good and bad. The manner in which I've tended to handle difficult times in my life is tied directly to the way I was brought up. Of course this is true of all of us. Our upbringing, the foundation of who we are, relates directly to how we come to perceive ourselves, what our expectations of ourselves are, and how we deal with the events that come our way. My upbringing was restrictive but also wonderful. I didn't feel short-changed, even when my parents put up barriers to the full expression of my free-spirited nature. But at the same time, I accepted the way things were because I felt I had no choice. Why fight a battle I knew I would lose?

It didn't help that before I lost all that weight, my father questioned everything I put into my mouth. He was concerned, as any parent would be, that I had gained so much weight in just three years—but for me, his nagging was just one more thing he was "getting on me" about. It seemed unfair. Wasn't I already the perfect kid? Didn't I obey him and my mother when they told me to do well in school, take care of the house, work in the family grocery store, not talk back, and always be respectful? Didn't I obey them when they told me I couldn't date, couldn't go to my American friends' parties, and couldn't stay out past nine p.m. even when I went to Arab friends' events?

In my last year of high school, I was invited to the senior prom by no fewer than five different guys. Two were from my own school, which meant they were an absolute "no way." The other three were Arab friends who wanted to take me to my prom even though they were already in college.

I ended up going with my third cousin. My father arranged it, although I didn't learn this until I went to pick my date up—he didn't have his driver's license yet. He confessed that he didn't actually want to go to my prom because he hadn't attended my school and wouldn't know anyone there. In fact, he bitched about it all the way to the hotel where the prom was being held. He even told me he wouldn't dance a single dance with me.

But as soon as we arrived he spotted a girl from his high school he knew and liked. She was there with one of our school's football players. All of a sudden my third cousin was begging me to dance. "Don't tell anyone we're cousins," he said. He wanted me to pretend he had brought me to the prom as a mercy date because I liked him so much!

"Take a hike," I said.

Later, one of my Arab friend's brothers (you still with me?) opened a nightclub for over eighteen year olds, and invited my group of friends to the opening. I dressed up in an amazing outfit: fitted black gauchos, a black vest lined with polyester silk, and a white ruffled blouse that gathered at the wrists and had a ruffled edge. My stomach was flat, my hair was feathered, and I was wearing my platform Famolare shoes (hey, it was 1976). I was so excited to go dancing at a club with my friends...until my dad told me I had to be home by nine o'clock.

Let me repeat: I was eighteen years old, and *my father told me I had to be home by nine*. In an Arab-American household, your age does not matter. If you live at home and you're an unmarried woman, you could be thirty and you'd still be expected home when your daddy tells you to be back. If that's nine p.m. then you make sure you're in the door at nine or earlier.

Still, I begged him to let me stay out later until he finally said, "Okay, you can leave at nine o'clock to be home by 9:30."

Guess what? I was home at 9:29. I didn't argue. Arguing would be useless.

That was one of the few times I wished I had older brothers. All my Arab girlfriends had older brothers, and they got to stay out as late as their brothers did because an older brother meant a dependable, trustworthy escort. Either that or they'd just sneak out at night like typical American teenagers, going secretly to clubs and having boyfriends.

Not me. On the one hand I was afraid about letting my parents down, and on the other I was afraid of getting caught. There was a third hand, too: I worried about ruining my reputation and therefore missing out on the life I wanted—which by then corresponded exactly with the life that was expected of me.

The fear of disappointing people—especially my parents—created a young woman who stifled her own feelings and regularly put others' desires first. Even now I'm famous amongst my friends for saying "Everything will be okay." And things *do* have a way of working out—but still, sometimes when I say those words it's just a way to soothe my own pain. Some things about yourself you cannot change unless you first change the way you handle those things.

Keep this in mind.

So we've figured out that as a young girl I overate partly out of rebellion and partly out of frustration. While my family life was filled with fun, love and passion, there was also, on a day-to-day level, the aggravation of being stuck in an Old World way of thinking.

But I got past it, right? After all, I did lose fifty pounds, become attractive, and enjoy high school. Everything was fine, really. I had no reason to slide back down into bad eating habits...right?

Wrong.

Weight Watchers has a slogan: "Nothing tastes as good as thin feels." But if that's true, why isn't feeling thin always enough to make us stay thin?

When you lose a lot of weight, there's an ironic side-effect: you really notice the difference between how you're treated when you're thin versus when you were fat. When I'm thin, men open doors for me with a look of admiration and appreciation—okay, I'll just say it: with lust—on their faces. But when I'm fat, if they open doors at all (notice I say *if*), they do so only because their mamas brought them up right. This internal split can create a part within us that rebels at the injustice. After all, everyone wants to be loved for who they are no matter their size.

As a youngster, being fat *and* being nagged about it made me feel both unlovable and like a failure. Even my parents seemed disgusted by me. Maybe they were afraid no one would want to marry me. That was what I thought at the time, although later I would learn that this wasn't the case at all: my parents nagged me out of simple concern and love. But at the time all I could think was: *If my folks feel this way about me, why should the rest of the world feel any differently?*

To make matters worse, in the years that I was fat I was told all the time—and I mean *all* the time—"You have such a pretty face. If only you'd lose weight."

Rebel? Yep, I wanted to...but how? Drugs and sex were out; my dad and mom would kill me and then disown me. I was too young to gamble. Even alcohol was out—as far as my parents were concerned, booze was as bad as drugs and sex.

So what's a girl to do when she feels like a failure, unlovable, and is, on top of that, fat? What's a girl to do when she needs to rebel but doesn't want to get herself killed or let anyone else down?

She eats, that's what.

It's a self-destructive cycle, the reverse of the one where moving leads to eating less leads to moving more. In this downward cycle, feeling worthless unless you're a certain weight leads to using food to deal with your bad feelings, which leads to gaining weight, which leads to feeling more worthless....

Each night before I go to sleep I agonize about my weight, and about losing weight, and about controlling my weight. I agonize about the same things when I wake up. The cycle is endless, constant. Battling your weight can overshadow every other problem in your life, even problems that should probably be at the forefront of your mind.

The messages we carry with us throughout our lives need to be tempered with the reality that comes with maturity and the ability to tell the difference between messages and reality. Some messages serve us well. But when they don't, it's time to take a hard look at the way we think, and make the changes necessary to live a healthier life in a healthier frame of mind.

No one is home when she gets back from school. Great! She has the place to herself: a rare event.

What sounds good? Chocolate, of course!

She walks to the buffet in the dining room where she knows her mother keeps the Sees Chocolates. She looks around to make absolutely sure no one else is around; sometimes her cousins or aunts and uncles drop by unexpectedly.

She pulls out the box and opens it. She'll have to select only two pieces, otherwise her mother might notice. Damn! Someone's already eaten her favorites. Probably one of her brothers. Her favorites are also theirs.

Finally she picks out two alternatives and rearranges the rest so the gaps will not be so noticeable. There. She puts the box carefully back where she found it.

The milk chocolate liquefies in her mouth. She savors each piece, the chocolate sticking to her teeth as she makes the pleasure last as long as possible.

She hopes her mother won't notice the missing pieces, but fears the worst. Somehow Mom always seems to know.

Oh well. If she gets in trouble, it will be worth it.

Milk chocolate....

DREAM A LITTLE DREAM

CHAPTER 5

*S*he pulls up to the drive-through window at Kentucky Fried Chicken and places an order for wings slathered in barbeque sauce, along with mashed potatoes and gravy and a buttered, honeyed biscuit. She knows she shouldn't be eating all that; she's on her way home for a big family dinner.

But that's fine. If she consumes everything she just ordered she'll only be able to eat a little at dinner with her family. Many times her parents have wondered how she can possibly have a weight problem when they see her eat so little.

If they knew the truth, they would be so upset....

So now you know what my family life was like, how I began to gain weight as a child, and how as a teenager I lost over fifty pounds and kept it off for five years.

What you want to know now is, what happened after *that*? Why did you gain back not only all that hard-lost weight, but more than two hundred additional pounds?

The answer is simple: I got married.

My relationship with Adam Taylor was a result of the intersection of two things: my dreams and my heritage. As you'll recall, my family originated from one man who had five sons. When my clansmen immigrated to America, most of them wanted to reap the rewards of living in the United States without losing their old-world values and culture. They founded the Ramallah Federation, whose objectives are to educate, blend, and create an atmosphere of understanding between Americans and Arabs. The Federation also aims to teach Arab-American children born in the United States about their heritage.

Remember me mentioning the San Francisco convention? In almost every major city in the U.S., Ramallah descendants form a Ramallah Club under the Ramallah Federation umbrella. Each year a different city hosts the annual Ramallah Federation Convention, which is attended by anywhere from three thousand to over ten thousand people from all over the U.S. and sometimes the world.

These conventions are held on the first Wednesday after the Fourth of July and continue through the following Sunday. They provide an opportunity for members to spend time with family members they don't usually get to see, and provide wonderful activities during the day and dinner dances in the evenings.

In 1977 my father announced that he, my mother, my sister and I would be traveling to Washington, D.C. to attend that year's convention. He'd planned a six-week getaway that would include various additional stops, including one in Chicago to attend a family friend's wedding, as well as in New York, Pittsburgh, and Connecticut.

I didn't want to go. I begged to stay home even though I loved sightseeing in the nation's capital, shopping in New York City and visiting my beloved grandmother in Connecticut. In fact it would have been the trip of a lifetime for me—but I did not want to go.

Why not? Why would a nineteen year-old girl turn down such an opportunity? There must have been a real significant reason, right?

There was. His name was Tony.

The brother of one of my best friends, Tony was twenty-four years old and gorgeous, and I had it very bad for him. I was a smitten kitten, and knew he liked me too. To make things even better, he came from a nice Palestinian family, I adored his mother, and his sister and I were great friends. How could I possibly leave him for six weeks?

My father insisted I go on the trip. It was time to for me to "debut," and the convention was the perfect place for it.

Oh, did I mention that another purpose of Ramallah conventions was to introduce young Ramallah men to young Ramallah women in order to form marriage matches?

Please don't go into shock. I'm not talking about arranged marriages. The way it works is this: If a young man and woman meet and like each other, they tell their parents, who then determine if the other person comes from a good family. If the young man's family approves of the young woman and her family, the male's father will call the lady's father and ask for a visit.

Of course, the female's family accepts, and soon the male's family, possibly including uncles and aunts, arrives at the home of the female's family.

During this visit the female is watched by the male's family to see if and how she helps her mother serve *maza* (Arabic appetizers), followed by fruit, followed by coffee and sweets. If the female does not exhibit the qualities expected from a bride and wife, the male's family will not encourage the match. But if the men are satisfied that she's a good match for their family (notice I don't say "their son"; Arabs believe that when a couple marries they wed not only the individual but his or her family as well), they encourage their son to ask the female if she would like to go out for a cup of coffee while the families continue to visit.

Of course the couple is chaperoned by sisters and brothers on this excursion; there's no way in hell the couple will be left alone for any length of time.

This was the prospect I faced and dreaded—but I did what a good Arab daughter does: I got on the plane with my parents and my sister, Judy. My Godmother's son David met us at the airport in D.C. and drove us to our hotel, which was also where the convention was to be held.

I was in awe of the scenery on the drive to the hotel. I caught David looking at me in the rearview mirror as if I was crazy. I told him we didn't have so many trees in San Diego. Scattered palm trees, yes. Thick lush woods, no.

After checking into the hotel we registered for the convention. I was already having fun. You see, once I realized I had no choice but to go on this trip, in my usual fashion I embraced the experience and determined to make the most of it.

That evening my mother and I dressed in our evening gowns—looking quite beautiful, if I say so myself—and walked to the head of the staircase that led down to the two ballrooms where there would be dinner, speeches, and, later, dancing to both Arab and American music, one type of music in each room.

But at the top of the stairs I froze. My mother, already a few steps down, turned to see what was holding me up. When she saw my face she said, "Linda, what's wrong?"

"Mom, do you remember me telling you about the recurring dream I have about a man standing at the end of a staircase and waiting for me to come down to him? Do you remember me describing that man to you?"

"Yes, what about it?"

"There he is. That's the man I'm supposed to marry."

My mother turned, looked, then walked back up to me. "Linda, you cannot marry him. He's your god-mother's son, and in the Syrian Orthodox church, the children of your godparents are considered the same as your blood brothers and sisters."

I couldn't believe it. There he stood: the man I had been awaiting for my entire life; the man I *knew* I was supposed to marry...and my mother was telling me it was impossible because of our religion.

As the cosmos would have it (the Arabs say *il naseeb*, which means "destiny"), Adam had noticed me as well, and told his mother he was interested in me. Of course, she also informed him that nothing could happen between us because I was her goddaughter.

The message couldn't be clearer, so Adam and I both accepted it. Nevertheless we were drawn to each other like magnets, and for the rest of the convention were inseparable. Every time I turned around, there he was. He even asked my father's permission to escort me to a room party being thrown by some of the Ramallah kids—and shockingly (I do mean I went into shock), my dad said, "Yes."

After the convention, Adam's parents invited us to come stay at their home in Virginia. During the three days we were there, the magnetic attraction between Adam and me only got stronger, even though we knew nothing could ever come of it.

I tried to put Adam out of my mind as my family and I moved on to the other places on our itinerary. I hadn't been very successful six weeks later when we arrived in Connecticut to visit my grandmother Annie. One morning I woke as my mother came into the bedroom trailed by my sister and grandmother. They all had huge grins on their faces. Only my father was missing; he had returned to California because someone had set fire to our grocery store (it turned out to be the butcher, who had apparently gone crazy one night. Maybe my brother had slingshot his backside with one pistachio shell too many).

I rubbed my eyes. "What's going on?"

"Linda," my mother said, "who did you see on this trip that you were interested in enough to marry?"

"Mom, I met lots of guys. Why, is someone asking for me? Who?"

"Who did you like the most?"

"Maaaaaaahm, who asked for me?"

"Tell me who you liked the most."

"Adam, but it can't be him."

My mom started to nod, a huge grin on her face.

I sat up. "Mom, it can't be. You said our church wouldn't allow it."

"Apparently the rules have changed. His family checked into it. They want us to fly down to Virginia and spend a few more days with them to see how you and Adam like each other."

To say I was elated would be an understatement. From the time I was a little girl my dreams had assured me that Adam and I were supposed to be together.

We spent another three days at his parent's home. One night he and I went out for dinner...along with three other couples: his brother, Paul, and his soon-to-be fiancé Mary; his cousin, Hesam, and his wife Reema; and his brother, Ned, and his date.

At the restaurant everyone except me ordered drinks. I was underage. They were all shocked that I had never had a drink, and Adam ordered me a Pina Colada. It was good.

After we left the restaurant Adam and I drove back to his parent's home, pulled into the circular drive-way and parked. Unchaperoned for once, we sat in his Corvette and talked about things that were important to both of us.

Finally we decided to take the conversation into the house. The moment Adam unlocked the front door we found ourselves staring at Adam's father, with his mother a few feet behind. My mother and sister stood at the top of the spiral staircase, my sister looking worried, and my mother furious.

Questions bombarded us. "Where were you? Do you realize it is two a.m.? Adam, how dare you keep her out this late! Linda, get up here immediately! Right now! Adam, what were you doing sitting in the car?"

Our answers stumbled over one another. "We were just talking. We didn't realize how late it was. Nothing happened. Yes, Mom! I'm coming!"

I ran up the steps, and my mother took me into the bedroom and shut the door behind her. She turned to me. "Nothing happened? You were just talking?"

"Yes, Mom."

Her face softened. "Well...did you have a good time?"

"I had a wonderful time."

The next morning Adam and I said good-bye again. His father asked me how I liked Virginia, and of course I answered that I loved the state.

"Good," he said.

Five days later, he called my father in San Diego and asked for permission for his son to marry me. My father asked me what I wanted, and of course I said yes.

Adam and I were married five months later, and the dream ended.

Perhaps I should have foreseen problems even before the wedding. One night my mother gave me wedding advice as we sat in her bedroom sharing a few tears. I had never been away from my family except for five days when I attended sixth grade camp, and now I would be flying across the country to live in Virginia.

Mom took me by the shoulders and looked into my eyes. "Don't worry about your wedding night," she said. "Just lie there and spread your legs open. He'll know what to do."

All I wanted to say was, "*Eeeeeew*!"

But then Mom said something that proved to be far more important. "Watch your weight. These people are all about appearances. They won't like it if you gain weight. Your future sister-in-law, Mary, is very thin; you'll look like Laurel and Hardy next to each other if you get fat."

There it was: even on my wedding day, even after five years of hard-preserved thinness, my weight was still an issue. In my parent's eyes I remained a potential fatty.

Was that all anyone ever focused on?

Adam and I married on January 29, 1978. Not long afterward my parents came to Virginia to attend Paul and Mary's wedding and to see me. The moment they saw me they looked concerned: I had gained ten pounds.

My in-laws were not happy about it, either. My mother-in-law wanted me to wear a certain gown to her son's wedding, but when I tried it on, the zipper would barely go up.

She told my mother she wouldn't blame Adam if he cheated on me. Can you imagine?

As for my husband, he never said anything about my weight—but then, within the first two months of our marriage—before I'd gained an ounce—he'd lost interest in sex, if not in me.

After that, with every passing day he became more cold and distant. I didn't know what to do. I wasn't used to rejection. I didn't know how to deal with it. Worse, I was lonely, with no family or friends nearby. I had a lot of time on my hands, so I kept an immaculate home...and learned to cook really well.

And there in the kitchen I made all my own friends: the foods I loved.

It also turned out that I was very fertile. As rarely as Adam and I had sex, I seemed to get pregnant every time. Still, even after four children, my relationship with my husband continued to grow only more distant. He was simply not interested—not in me, not in our children, not in our family.

Yet I loved him still, the man of my dreams. And everything always works out, right? I certainly wanted and intended for my marriage to prosper. But the more rejection I felt, the more I ate, and the more I ate the more weight I gained, and the more weight I gained the more rejection I felt. The cycle was vicious, and all along the way I could hear my mother-in-law's words in the back of my head: "I wouldn't blame Adam for cheating on her if she gets fat."

So I got fat. I tried to lose weight, but after dropping twenty or thirty pounds I'd put it all back on again, and then some. I struggled every day, and every day I failed. When my marriage finally ended after thirteen years, I had gained over two hundred and twenty-five pounds.

My family helped me through the ugly divorce that followed. The details are unimportant except for the fact that by the time I returned to California I was an emotional and economic wreck.

To make matters worse, I left Virginia with only three of my children, the youngest. By an arrangement between my father, my soon-to-be ex-husband, his father and uncle, Adam retained custody of my oldest son, Steven. According to my father, this was the best way because Steven didn't want to come to California; he didn't even want to be told when the rest of us were leaving. He preferred to find out we were gone when Adam picked him up from school. If he ever changed his mind about coming to live with me, I was told, he would be flown out to California.

In a way I understood all this. Steven had already made it clear he didn't care for my father, who he was convinced was the instigator of the problems in our marriage: "Your mother hero-worships him," Adam had told him.

And he was right: I did hero-worship my father. It was my father who had always been there for me, and he was still there the day I left my loveless marriage. The point is, I sincerely believed that by leaving my eldest son with his father, I was doing the right thing. I feared he would run away if I tried to bring him to the West coast with me. I certainly didn't question the claim that Steven didn't even want to be told when the rest of us left for California.

Still, the moment I arrived in the Golden State I called my son to make sure he was okay, and to ask, again, if he'd like to fly out and join us after all.

"No." Steven's voice shocked me: it was as cold as Adam's. "You abandoned me. You didn't even let me say goodbye. I hate you."

That happened over twenty-four years ago. It took years of calling Steven, talking to him, and being there for him even from a distance of three thousand miles before he regained his trust in me and my love for him. As for me, I still feel the pain and guilt I felt at that time. I am his mother, and no matter what actually happened between Adam and my father, I should have told Steven how badly I wanted him to come to California with me. Had he refused, at least it would have been his decision based on real information.

In later years he told me that he chose to stay with his father for two reasons: he didn't like my dad, and he believed that if he stayed he would be treated like an only child and given more of the things he wanted.

I shook my head. "I don't believe you. You love your brothers and sister too much for that."

He looked down. "You're right. The real reason I stayed was that I knew you'd always be there for me, no matter how far apart we were. But Dad...I was afraid if I traveled too far away from him it would be like, 'Out of sight, out of mind.'"

Sadly, this perception proved to be accurate—and not just for Steven. Adam was never there for any of his children; he didn't even pay a cent of child or spousal support.

Looking back, I can see that when I married Adam and found his family so negative and condescending, I should have stood up for myself. I should have told all of them, including Adam, that the way they treated me was hurtful and disrespectful. Instead, I tried to be diplomatic. I wanted our relationships to go smoothly. But as one of my sister's friends says, "You have to teach people how you want to be treated. If you allow them to treat you like a doormat, you'll become a doormat."

She's right. I became a doormat. For thirteen years I let Adam and his family walk all over me, and I stuffed down my resentment and sadness by stuffing food down my throat. For me, food was comforting. Food was the only thing in my life I could control. No one could tell me what to eat, what not to eat, or how much to eat. I would show them!

Instead, of course, I showed myself.

She looks at the clock. The kids will be in school for another three hours, and Domino's Pizza delivers. She places the call for a large pepperoni pie.

When the pizza arrives she sits down to devour it while watching her favorite soap opera, The Young and The Restless. *The melted cheese mixing with the sweet tomato sauce tastes so good....*

For the next thirty minutes she doesn't think about how frustrated she is that her husband never comes home until everyone else had gone to sleep. She doesn't think about how unhappy she is in her marriage. She doesn't think about how she'll survive if she asks for a divorce.

No: the time is dedicated to forgetting, and the only way to forget is to devour her pizza and wash it down with ice-cold cans of Diet Pepsi.

After she's done she puts the remnants of the pizza into a large trash bag and seals it tight.

Time to pick the kids up from school. She drives to the shopping center nearest the school, parks beside a dumpster and throws in the trash bag containing the evidence of her addiction. Then she gets the kids, takes them home and serves them a snack.

While they watch television she prepares a fabulous dinner.

Which she will eat, too, of course.

WOULDA-SHOULDA-COULDA

CHAPTER 6

The tears roll down her cheeks as she sits in her car. Her heart aches and aches. She doesn't know how to express her agony. Words like Failure! *and* Get yourself together, for God's sake! *scream at her from her mind.*

She closes her eyes and prays. "God, help me. Help me, please. It's not supposed to be like this. I miss my son. Please make him understand I want him with me and always have, and let him feel how much I love him. Please, God...please help me!"

She wipes the tears from her cheeks, tilts down the mirror on the visor and examines her face. Then she pulls her makeup bag out of her purse, quickly fixes her face and glances around to make sure no one witnessed her mini-breakdown.

"Stop this crap," she tells herself. "Enough is enough."

When she twists the ignition key, the CD player

switches on and Donna Summer's "Last Dance" blares from the speakers. She loves her music loud.

She starts to drive home. After going a few blocks, and without conscious thought, she turns the car into the parking lot of her favorite Italian restaurant. She parks and walks inside. When she comes back out she's carrying a giant slice of pepperoni pizza.

Also a meatball sub, a side of fries, and a large Diet Coke.

NOW she can go home.

As pathetic as it sounds, that was me after I returned to San Diego. As quickly as I told myself to knock it off was exactly how quickly I'd go out and get more food. I just couldn't seem to help myself.

Food made me feel better. More specifically, this particular *kind* of food—rich, caloric, and satisfying—helped me sleep, and only when I was asleep did I not feel emotional pain. (I'm not ordinarily much of a sleeper even at the best of times. I'm lucky to get more than four to five hours a night.)

You'd think that returning to San Diego and the supporting arms of my family and friends would have comforted me. And to a degree it did—but not enough to stop me from feeling like a failure. Although I tried to keep my happy face on all the time, I was not happy—and pretending that I was happy was painful. In reality I had only seven hundred dollars to my name and three children to support.

On top of that I had to face everyone in my family and the Arab community with my shame. People asked unbelievable questions about my divorce. They seemed especially interested in finding out what drove me to leave my husband, and if all the horrible rumors they had heard about my marriage were true.

I answered as best I could, and tried to return to the life I had led before I married Adam. I returned to my church and became a Sunday school teacher. I led the youth group. I made new friends. I also became the office manager of my brother's dental practice. That, at least, was a perfect arrangement. My mother had been his office manager for years, and wanted to retire—plus my dad wanted her back home with him.

Plus, I needed a job.

I'm proud to say that twenty-two years later I'm very good at what I do. I've been an integral part of helping my brother grow a successful dental practice, and I love making a difference in our patients' lives. I'm also the self-proclaimed Rocky Balboa of fighting insurance companies—and winning. So that part of my life feels great.

But when I first came home, *nothing* felt great. There was the divorce, and the way I'd left my eldest son behind. There was my financial situation, and having to live with my parents again. And on top of all that was the fact that I'd left home weighing one hundred and fifty pounds and returned at over four hundred pounds. When I looked at my parents I wondered what they thought of me. They knew my husband had had no real regard for me, but still, perhaps they believed my marriage would have survived had I not gained any weight. Hadn't my mother warned me about exactly that?

We all had to make adjustments to our new lives. My kids had to acclimate to the breakup of their parents and to the absence of their eldest brother. They had to adjust to the rules of my parent's home, which, while not terribly different from my own, were not identical. And my parents had to readjust to having kids in the house after years of being on their own, not to mention dealing with a grown daughter who was falling apart.

My joining the workforce was another adjustment. I'd always planned to be a stay-at-home mom, raising my children and participating in all their school and extracurricular activities. Now I had to leave the kids in the care of my parents while I went off to work. God bless my mom and dad. Sometimes I think they slipped into the new situation better than I did, although at times it was the clash of two worlds. To say that my kids were active would be an understatement, and to say that my dad wanted peace and quiet would be accurate.

Still, we all not only survived, we did well together—until my children approached their teens, when it became clear that the time had come for us to strike out on our own.

By then I was ready to go. I wanted to set an example for my kids. I wanted them to know that while it's all right to accept help from others when you have real need, at some point you must take responsibility for the life you've chosen.

My first apartment had two bedrooms, two bathrooms, kitchen, dining room, living room, deck, and one parking space. Best, it was all mine (as long as I paid the rent, of course).

We moved in. Nick and Tommy shared one room while Nadia and I shared the other. I felt especially bad for my daughter, stuck in a room with her mother. Instead of girly teenage things and posters on the walls, she had Mom's Wedgewood and Ainsley pieces and an elegant bedspread with shams. She and I even had to share a bed.

But Nadia never complained. She knew we were doing the best we could. And honestly, sharing a bed was fun. She'd tell me her secrets, and we'd giggle until it was time to go to sleep.

Thankfully the boys also got along well and didn't fight much. Still, to say we had no problems would be a lie. Typical teenage rebellion invaded my home like it does anyone else's. On top of that there was the financial struggle. Making it from month to month was tough, even after my daughter got a job and started helping as much as she could.

Have you heard people say, "As hard as it was, it was the best time of our lives?" In a way those words fit our situation. We relied on each other, my kids and I, and together kept our family together through all the ups and downs.

But at one point during this period my father asked me if I was happy.

"Because if you are," he said, "you should be losing weight."

Well, I wasn't losing weight; not an ounce—and no, I was not happy. Even though my kids and I were doing all right, I still felt incessantly guilty about the divorce; I still felt as if I had let my both my children and my parents down.

In other words, I was living in a woulda-shoulda-coulda world. I woulda done things differently if I had another chance; I shoulda had a great marriage; we coulda fixed our marriage if only…

Was I ever going to get over it?

Nine years went by, then ten, eleven—and I was still stuck in the past, struggling through the darkness of my divorce and the lack of respect my ex-husband had showed me and our children. I couldn't seem to let it go.

But I hid my pain from the rest of the world—except for my best friend, Sandie. She knew everything I felt, including how much the divorce still affected me. She was the only person I could completely confide in. She still is. Sandie never judges me. She'll chastise me, especially if I'm coming down too hard on myself, but she has a way of always seeing the very best in me.

At least now that I was living on my own I no longer had to sneak-eat. If I wanted to gobble down junk food, there was no one around to give me The Look. You know The Look I'm talking about: judgmental, disapproving, yet somehow meant to encourage you to not self-destruct. Well, now that I lived in my own place I could self-destruct if I wanted to, and that was that.

Of course, that aspect of my new-found freedom set a bad example for my children. Don't misunderstand. It's not like I was sitting around day after day eating nothing but junk food—on the contrary, most of the time I was trying to lose weight and was even successful a couple of times. For six months I stuck to the Phase One Induction Plan of the Atkins diet, lost seventy-two pounds and felt incredible. Although I still weighed in the three hundreds, after pushing 430 pounds, I found that 300-anything felt like 125 pounds of greatness.

Next I joined Kaiser Permanente's Optifast program and lost over ninety pounds in three months.

The lesson was this: I could stick to a diet for a good period of time, but then something would trigger a meltdown inside me and I'd put the weight right back on again—along with some extra for good measure.

My children were worried about me; in fact they were terrified they'd wake one morning and find me dead. Occasionally they rallied together to do an "intervention": They would tell me how concerned they were about me, remind me of the bad habits I was teaching them, point out that I needed to set a good example. Then they would cry and tell me how much they loved me and that they couldn't bear it if something happened to me.

So the next day I'd start a new diet. I'd begin exercising again. And the program would last as long as it was going to last, but not one day longer.

Then there was the matter of men. From time to time I'd meet someone I really liked. Sandie and I enjoyed going out dancing. Sometimes on these excursions we'd meet men and dance with them, but things never went any further. Men—fat or thin—have always been attracted to me. I'm told it's because I have bedroom eyes, I'm a good flirt, I'm nice, and I'm funny. But I didn't believe that at my weight I would be taken seriously as a potential lover or wife by any man. When a man told me I was beautiful he invariably added that I should lose weight. Then he'd go ask the skinny girl to dance, and spend the rest of the evening with her.

Clearly, if I wanted to meet a nice man and build a new life, I had to get my exterior looking as hot as my interior felt.

Meanwhile, for myself I wanted a man who was nice, hardworking, respectful, funny, and generous of self—meaning willing to share himself and his life with me and mine. I wanted someone intelligent and down to earth. He had to love children and show that he could be a good father figure for my kids. And he had to love me for who I was no matter my size.

I knew that such men were out there somewhere; I just hadn't found one yet. Not that I seemed to be meeting anyone else's criteria either.

But I didn't worry about it. When I went out, I truly went just to dance and have fun with my friends. If I happened to meet a man, great. If not, I was fine with that, too. After all, the rest of my time was plenty busy with me trying to take care of my brother's office, raise three kids, and meet other family obligations. Relationships need time to develop, and for me, time was a luxury. I worked at my brother's practice every day, sometimes half-days on weekends. My son, Nick, surfed and needed rides to the beach (I loved watching him surf. We shared a spiritual connection with the ocean, whose enormity somehow brought us closer to God. We got this about each other). Nadia—God bless her—worked full time at Little Caesar's Pizza while also attending school full time. She helped carry the financial load of our family. Tommy was a musician who played in three different bands in his high school, in two bands he and his friends had put together, and also in the Palomar College band.

Every night after work I'd pick Tommy up from one rehearsal and take him to another rehearsal or a gig. Then I'd clean house, shop, cook, have family and friends over, or go to visit them. On top of that, for two years I was Band Booster President. Yeah, you might say I was busy.

And that was fine; I loved my new life with my family. The only thing it needed to make it perfect was to have my eldest son with us. By then Steven was in his teens and, from what I could find out, having trouble with both his father and his stepmother. Still, he didn't want to come live with us in California.

At times I was still overtaken by guilt about him. On these occasions you might find me sitting in my car in an isolated parking lot, devouring a giant slice of pizza, a meatball sub and an order of fries. I couldn't eat all that food, but I'd consume part of the pizza, and the meatballs dripping with melted provolone, and some fries drenched in ketchup. All washed down with Diet Coke, which erases calories, right?

I simply didn't deal well with guilt or emotional upheavals, so I ate my way to numbness even as some part of me screamed from an almost-sound-proofed room, *"Stop! Don't eat that! Don't give in!"*

With each bite I swallowed, that voice of reason grew fainter and fainter... until I couldn't hear it at all.

She called her ex-husband to discuss some of the problems Steven had told her he was having with his father. Such conversations always ended with her pleading with Adam to show an interest in not only Steven but the rest of his children as well. She told him how hurt they were that he never called them, never sent birthday cards, and rarely sent Christmas cards, let alone gifts.

He always promised the same things: He would call them. He would start sending child support payments.

She knew he would do nothing.

Finally she hung up. Her heart ached. Her ex seemed to have no comprehension of what he was doing to his children, how he was harming their souls, the pain he was causing them all.

She made her way to the kitchen. After cooking up a pound of spaghetti and a quick sauce, she sat down and ate two huge helpings. With each swallow the knot in her throat pained her more, but she forced the food down.

With tears stinging her cheeks, she ate more and more.

ANGELS IN THE CORNER

*S*he's made up her mind: today is the day she'll start her new diet. She'll begin by emptying out the cupboards, the refrigerator, and all her stashes.

She starts in the kitchen with the baked goods. Cookies go straight into the garbage, followed by chips and candy. She reaches for a huge milk chocolate bar. Looks at it for a moment. Begins to tear off the wrapper.

Nope! Out it goes. She won't allow junk food to rule her life and ruin her health; not anymore.

She feels proud of herself, and even gives a little laugh. How ridiculous that a chocolate bar has so much power over her! She laughs again and silently calls herself a dork.

Next she opens the refrigerator and throws out the leftover lasagna and garlic bread. That's especially difficult to do. Thankfully there isn't enough lasagna left to freeze, so she doesn't feel quite so bad.

Speaking of the freezer, that comes next. She opens the container of ice cream. Good! Someone else has already gotten to it, leaving it almost empty. Out, out, out it goes!

Now it's time to face her secret stashes. In her bedroom she opens her sock drawer. In the back, under the socks she never wears, are two candy bars. Straight into the garbage they go.

She ties the garbage bag shut and heads out the door to her car. She unlocks it, opens the console and grabs a bag of jellybeans. Then she walks to the Dumpster and throws in both the garbage and the candy.

As she turns and walks back into her home she feels a surge of pride.

But she's also sad. How did she ever allow herself to get to the point where she has to rid her home entirely of sugar?

She stops that line of thinking.

"No negativity!" she says out loud. "I can do this."

In fact, at that moment she believes she can do anything.

She's wrong.

After the house cleansing I was hell-bent on losing weight—and keeping it off this time. By that point my kids and I had been living on our own for three years, and our life together, overall, was pretty good. Although Nick gave me a hard time with typical teen-age rebellion, Nadia was working hard and attending community college on a scholarship, and Tommy, not yet sixteen, was busy with school and all the bands he played in. By then Steven was out of Adam's house and living on his own, traveling the country building cell towers. He'd become close with a girl, Lauren, whom I had not yet met but could tell was very important to him. So my eldest son was happy, doing well financially, all grown up.

One fine summer day, Nadia, Tommy and I were playing around in the swimming pool of our apartment complex when Nadia said, "Mom, do you promise not to get mad if I tell you something?"

That was my Nadia. She'd do something she knew would make me livid, then wait to tell me until she knew that no matter what happened, I just couldn't get angry.

She admitted that she'd lied to me about spending the night recently at the house of a friend. The friend had lied, too, telling her grandmother she would be sleeping at our home. In reality, both girls had gone to a nightclub in Tijuana. Later, as they were leaving the club, two Mexican police officers had stopped them and given them a very rough time. Nadia swore she would never go to T.J. again.

Of course I was grateful that she was there in the swimming pool with me, healthy, laughing, and unharmed. Still, although I couldn't really get mad, I could and did give her a solid lecture about all the horrible things that could have happened to an underage young lady down there across the border. But I was pretty sure the encounter with the *Federales* had, on its own, frightened her enough to serve as both deterrent and punishment.

So that was our life. We all worked hard, and when we had time together we enjoyed our simple existence.

On November 1, shortly after his sixteenth birthday, Tommy caught a cold. This was a first: Tommy never got colds.

After a week, when he didn't feel better, I made an appointment with his pediatrician. Nadia took him to the appointment for me. The doctor said Tommy had a bad cold, that was all—a viral thing that antibiotics couldn't help—and sent them home.

A week later Tommy was no better; in fact he was coughing more and more often, seemed exhausted, and was having trouble breathing. This time I personally took him to the doctor. Again we were sent home with the assurance that Tommy was suffering from nothing worse than a bad chest cold, and required only rest and fluids.

The following week Steven called to tell us he was working in Las Vegas. Lauren had come to visit him, and they wanted to drive to California to see us and so we could meet Lauren. The problem was, they didn't have a car.

God bless Nick. He drove to Vegas, gathered the couple up and brought them back to San Diego, making the round trip in about nine hours.

As soon as I saw Lauren, I loved her. She was beautiful, with the sweetest heart, and it was obvious she and Steven were crazy about each other.

We stayed up all night, and I had to shut the windows because we got to laughing so loud and so hard. Tommy's lingering cold didn't stop him from joining in on the fun. He even went with us the next day to the Fashion Valley mall for shopping, and out to dinner at an all-you-can-eat Chinese buffet that served crab legs. In my happiness I kept my appetite under control with little effort.

My happiness inflated to euphoria when Steven announced that he and Lauren were engaged to marry. When the cries of joy died down he shared how he had popped the question. He'd picked her up from work and told her they were driving to the shopping mall where their friend worked at a movie theater. He'd parked under the marquee on the street and escorted Lauren out of his car—then got down on one knee and pointed up at the marquee. It read, "Lauren, will you marry me?"

She'd said yes.

When their visit ended I found it hard to take them to the airport and say goodbye. They were going to marry on March sixteenth, 2002; we had a wedding to plan for.

In the meantime Tommy's cold just kept getting worse. During November and December I took him to the doctor's office five times. More than once I found him coughing up blood, and rushed him to the emergency room where his pulse was found to be over 220 beats per minute. The ER doctors gave him breathing treatments—his cold, they said, had turned into viral bronchitis. No medicine would help him.

I was getting more and more worried. Tommy's condition was so bad he couldn't go to school; he couldn't even sleep without coughing. I'd find him kneeling on the floor with his elbow propped on the mattress and his head cradled in the palm of his hand. He wanted to get better because he missed playing in his bands.

Also, we'd planned our first vacation as a family since my divorce twelve years before: we would be joining my parents, brothers and sister and their families for a trip to Las Vegas without my father paying our way. In fact, even though most of the family would leave Vegas after two days, Nadia, Tommy, and I planned to stay for five.

Instead, I found myself tempted to cancel the trip entirely. Tommy did not seem to be getting better. Although he pleaded with me to continue with the original plan, I first took him back to see his doctor.

"He can go to Vegas," the doctor said, "provided he keeps things low-key."

I wanted to make this a very special trip. Tommy was into magic as well as music, and was very good at performing tricks, so I bought us tickets to see David Copperfield. By that time Tommy had lost his voice. He seemed extremely weak, and was not even interested in eating anymore (and Mislehs are *never* not interested in eating). We cut the trip short and drove home.

On the first Saturday of January, 2002, I parked my car in the lot across from the medical offices. During the walk across the street, Tommy had to stop every few steps to catch his breath, and I made up my mind: we would not be leaving that building until the doctor did something to make my son better.

Tommy's regular doctor was not on duty so we saw someone else, a woman. She listened to my son's chest and told me she thought he had pneumonia. To make sure, she arranged for us to walk over to the hospital for a chest x-ray.

"I'm sure you won't have to come back over here again," she said confidently. "After the radiologist confirms my diagnosis I'll call in a prescription at the hospital pharmacy, so you'll be right there to pick it up."

We crept across to the radiology department at the hospital, stopping repeatedly for Tommy to catch his breath. I'd offered to get him a wheelchair, but he'd refused.

"I can walk that far, Mom."

After the x-rays were taken we sat in the waiting room and waited for the doctor to call and tell us to go to the pharmacy. A half hour passed. An hour. An hour and half. And still we waited.

Finally the receptionist called us to the desk. "The doctor would like you to go back to her office," he said.

I looked at Tommy's pale face and shook my head. "She said she'd call a prescription in to the pharmacy here. We're supposed to fill it and go home."

"I'm sorry, ma'am, but the doctor was insistent. You have to go back to her office."

So we did. By the time we got there everyone except the doctor herself had gone home for the day. She sat down next to Tommy, and I sat across from them. She pulled his chest x-ray out of a folder. I looked at it in confusion. I'd seen many chest x-rays in my life, and there was something very wrong with this one.

"Where are his lungs?" I said. "And what is that huge mass in his chest?"

The doctor looked at me. "Ms. Misleh, that's Tommy's heart."

I stared at her, confused. The human heart is the size of a fist. This one seemed to take up my son's entire chest cavity.

She said, "The cold virus Tommy's been fighting for so long attacked his heart and caused it to enlarge."

I could see that for myself: in the x-ray my son's heart was as large as a four-month old baby. It was so big his lungs weren't even visible.

"Your son has congestive heart failure due to cardiomyopathy," the doctor said.

I felt my own heart pounding wildly. "What does that mean?"

"It means Tommy has to be admitted to the hospital right away. It means...he needs a heart transplant."

I sat frozen in my seat, in shock and unsure of what to do. I looked at Tommy. He did not seem to have a reaction; then I realized it simply took too much effort at that moment for him to feel anything. He was too sick to register a response. Truth be told, he looked as if death might be welcome. He was too exhausted to care.

The doctor told us she'd already made arrangements to admit Tommy into intensive care under the care of her husband, Dr. Cocalis, a renowned heart specialist.

"Is there anyone you want to call?" she asked.

Despite my terror, I gathered my wits and started phoning my parents, my brother, my daughter, and my other sons. Steven was too busy with his work and wedding plans to come to California at that time. I told him it was okay; the doctors were trying to stabilize Tommy, but if things got worse I'd find a way to make sure Steven got out to San Diego.

Then I called Adam and informed him of everything that was happening. My conclusion was, "You might want to make plans to come out here."

There was a pause. "If Tommy gets really bad, I'll come."

What? If Tommy gets *really* bad? I'd just told the son of a bitch that his son was dying and needed a heart transplant—assuming a suitable heart could be found—and his response was that he'd come *if Tommy got really bad?*

Everyone else met us at the hospital, where Tommy was admitted and given a thorough examination by Dr. Cocalis.

When the doctor came out of Tom's room he sat us down and told us exactly what we were facing. Tommy was dying. Without a heart transplant he *would* die. They'd keep him in intensive care for a while to try to stabilize him, and if they managed that they'd send him home—but he could not go to school and would need to take many medications just to stay alive until a suitable heart could be found.

Nick and Nadia contacted all of Tommy's friends, and within an hour over thirty kids, parents and family members crowded into the ICU waiting room. Since only two people at a time could go into Tommy's room, for the next several hours we took turns visiting him.

That evening, and every evening afterward, I stayed with Tommy in his room. A young nurse to whom I will be forever grateful made me a bed next to my son's. She even tucked me in.

Despite my last conversation with Adam, I called him periodically to give him updates. Why did I bother? What was wrong with me that I kept reaching out to a man who obviously didn't care at all about his children? Was I just stupid?

Tommy stayed in intensive care for six weeks. By mid-February he was stable enough to come home, although even then we made weekly trips back to see Dr. Cocalis.

Steven's wedding was set for the following month. Tommy wanted to attend, and Dr. Cocalis said the trip was possible...at a huge risk. It might be too much for Tommy; it might kill him. Tom was furious when I said he could not go. My mom offered to stay and take care of him so I could attend my oldest son's wedding.

I've often wondered if I made a mistake by not letting Tommy attend, too. After all, if his future was in limbo, shouldn't he be allowed to spend what might be his last days in whatever way he wanted?

No! If there was a chance, even a hope, that Tommy could recover from this situation, I had to preserve it. I refused to believe that he would not receive a new heart and go on with his life as before. I refused to believe he would not be fine, just fine.

Under the enormous weight of all this stress and doubt, I sometimes ate and sometimes didn't. If we had a good day at the hospital, I ate decently. If we had a bad day, I ate very little. But if we had a *very* bad day, the kind of day where I was afraid I might lose my son, I would eat terribly: pizza and candy bars, items easily accessible in the hospital cafeteria. The kind of foods that calm me down and raise my dopamine levels enough to numb me for a while.

During the next two years Tommy went back and forth to doctor appointments and for long stays at the hospital. A picc line was put into his arm to feed his heart the medicines it needed to keep him alive until a transplant became available. The bags arrived every other day, each at a cost of fifteen hundred dollars. Thank goodness for insurance.

Another thing to be thankful for: five months after Tommy's diagnosis, he and I moved into a rental home owned by my friend Paola. By then Nick had moved away to Pensacola, Florida. Our new house had four bedrooms, two baths, a large kitchen/dining area (woohoo!), a living room, a garage (woohoo!) and a nice back yard with a patio.

It had been twelve years since I'd lived in a house of my own (even though I was renting), and I loved it. *We* loved it. Nadia finally had a room of her own, and I let her decorate it any way she wanted. Tommy had his own room, too.

When Tommy was at home, he, Nadia and I made the most of our "new normal" life. We cherished our time together. Whenever Tommy returned to the hospital, that became the "new normal."

That was how we spent the next year and a half.

In August of 2003, Tommy started to fail. He was now seeing the cardiac team at the University of California, San Diego. The doctor in charge, Dr. Greenberg, told me they needed to find a heart soon; the meds were no longer enough to sustain my son's life.

I still had hope that the doctors would find a replacement heart and save Tommy. I conducted many conversations with God. I even had the audacity to yell at Him (privately, of course) to save my son, to heal him. I was angry. I wanted Tommy to live. My heart broke every time I saw the suffering he had to endure every day.

But Tommy never complained. Only once did he lose control.

I heard him crying in his room. Sobbing – angry, frustrated sobs, and my heart broke. He had been so strong. For me, he had been so strong.

I opened his door to comfort him.

"Get out! Get out!" he screamed.

"I'm only trying to help you. Don't yell at me!" I screamed back, my own anger and fear rising to the surface. There was nothing I could do to fix my son's heart, to save his life. I realize that now, although I couldn't see it then, nor could I allow myself to feel then my fury. I don't think I even knew *how* to recognize that kind of anger.

Tommy stood and stalked toward me, glaring, and suddenly everything I had been holding within me exploded. I found myself screaming at him as he was screaming at me. What we said, I no longer remember.

Nadia came running in. "Stop! Both of you stop!"

At that same moment Tommy wrapped his hands around my throat.

I spit in his face.

He blinked, and his hands dropped. We held one another and sobbed.

"I'm so tired of being strong for you, mom," he wept.

"I know. I know. Me too, Tommy. Me too. Please forgive me, son. Please forgive me."

Today I realize the explosion was natural. We were both so scared, so angry, and working so hard to keep ourselves together. But years would pass before I could deal with the guilt I felt for fighting with him that day.

Just before Tommy's eighteenth birthday, the doctors sat us down and told us they feared they would not get a transplant heart in time. If one did not become available within the next two to four weeks, the only solution would be to implant an artificial heart. That would buy Tommy a few more years at most—while simultaneously taking him off the transplant list until the artificial heart failed.

The next day, September fourth, Tommy turned eighteen. What a difference a day makes! At the stroke of midnight he became an adult, and the final decision about having an artificial heart implanted became his alone.

I wanted him to do it, but he refused. "If they can't find a transplant heart," he said, "I'm ready to go." He didn't want to continue living the way he had been for the past two years, only to go through the whole mess again when the artificial heart inevitably failed.

With each passing day he looked worse. I called Adam and told him what was going on.

My ex-husband's response: "They'll find a heart, and when he gets it, I'll come out."

Later I learned that for the past two years Adam and his parents had been telling people that Adam had been making monthly trips from Virginia to California to see his son, and that I was exaggerating the extent of Tommy's illness.

On October seventeenth, 2003, I was at work catching up on some things when I received a phone call from my mom.

"I've just been to see Tommy," she said. "He didn't look good, Linda. I'm worried."

Shortly after that my friend, Merryl, also called. She'd also just visited Tommy. Meryl held a special place in both my heart and my son's. More than once during the time Tommy was living at home she had picked him up, driven him to school and sneaked him into band class. Because of insurance liability he wasn't supposed to be there, but Merryl took him for the hour anyway and then brought him back home. Thank you, Merryl.

I told her I was on my way to the hospital. When I got there I parked by the rear entrance. The hospital security team knew that I came there every day and couldn't afford to park in the public lot, so they allowed me to leave my car by the rear entrance for free. The same was true of the hospital valet team, which would valet my car for free when I had to get into the hospital quickly. Remarkable people.

When I got to Tommy's room I was horrified by how he looked: ashen, struggling. Still, as usual, he kept his sense of humor and tried to make me laugh.

Twenty minutes later his phone rang. Tommy answered. The coolest cat ever, he kept saying "Okay... okay..." Then, "I'll see you soon."

He hung up. I asked him who it was. He shrugged.

"That was Stephanie, the transplant coordinator. I got a heart."

I didn't hug him. He was in too much pain for that. Instead I jumped up and down (imagine how hard that was for a four hundred pound woman), scream-ing, "We got a heart! We got a heart!"

Nurses and doctors came running to see what was wrong.

"Nothing! We got a heart!"

We all began to leap up and down. Tears streamed down my cheeks. Tommy told a nurse to get me a bed before I keeled over. Then, in his cool fashion, he started making calls to our family and friends to tell them the news. The one person Tommy didn't think to call was his father.

I'm the one who called Adam.

"I knew he'd get a heart," he said. But he was making no plans to come out to see his son. Had it been me, I would have been on the first plane I could book.

That evening Tommy was wheeled into surgery. My parents, my brother, Anton, Nadia and several of her co-workers, her boss Joe, and our dear friends the McCartys gathered together to wait the long hours ahead. The surgery was successful, and the next morning Tommy returned to intensive care to begin the healing and waiting process. We prayed that his body would accept the new heart.

Fourteen days later we all went home—an unheard-of recovery time, we were told.

But two days after that Tommy was back in the hospital, where he stayed until November 11. The next week and a half felt like an eternity as my son fought for his life. I witnessed him suffer through the horrible procedures needed to help his heart function.

God bless the cardiac team and the nurses. Oh God, please bless these people forever. They did everything they could to save my son.

On November 14, back home, he woke feeling unwell and had to return to the hospital yet again. The cardiac team examined him and said they'd call us that evening with the results of the latest blood tests, but they were not terribly concerned. "After all, he *is* recovering from open heart surgery."

We got home at three-thirty in the afternoon, and I started making dinner. At five o'clock the phone rang. The cardiac team reported that the tests had come back negative: as predicted, Tommy's lethargy appeared to be simply part of the recovery process.

The next day, Saturday, Tommy woke and told me he didn't feel well and wanted to stay in bed. When I asked him what he wanted for lunch and dinner, he chose Irish stew.

Throughout the day I looked in on him constantly. Every two hours he needed his blood pressure checked and his temperature taken, and he had to swallow a percentage of the sixty-five pills he was required to take each day.

When I brought him his stew he said he was too tired to eat, and I noticed that his legs kept sliding off the bed and dangling. I would pick them up, slip them back onto the bed and tuck them in. Before long they would slide off the bed again.

As the day went on Tommy began saying strange things. He told me that Dr. Hermann, one of his cardiologists, was standing in the room with a clipboard. I chalked it up to the effect of his pain meds.

Next he said there was an angel in the corner of the room.

"She's come for me," he said. "She looks beautiful, golden...."

As the day went on he described various relatives who had died but who were now in the room with him. I didn't want to believe what I was hearing; I went on telling myself it was the pain meds talking. I did call the cardiology department to report what he was experiencing and they agreed it must be the drugs.

Denial is such a powerful force. You just don't want to believe certain things. You ignore the signs—because if you face them, you'll realize you might have to give up something you value.

At midnight I went into Tommy's room to give him his meds and check his blood pressure and temperature. His temp was low, so I called the cardiology team member on call. He said to wait until three o'clock and check Tommy's temperature again. If it was any lower I was to bring him in immediately.

I went into my bedroom and set the alarm clock for two-thirty to make sure I was wide awake at three o'clock.

When I fell asleep I was gripped by the most terrifying dream. I was living in a beautiful house in a cul-de-sac. It was nighttime and I was in the garage with the rolling door open. I noticed that the house two doors down from mine, situated higher on the hillside, was all lit up. I heard music coming from it, and figured the neighbors were having a big party.

A limousine pulled up in front of my driveway and my three aunts stepped out. All of them were dressed in black from head to toe. At first I thought they were going to the party at the neighbor's home, then I looked from one face to the other and realized how sad they all looked.

"Why are you here?" I asked.

"We're here for you. To be with you."

"With me? Why would you need to be with..."

And then it hit me. My Aunt Jamileh had lost her son, Steve, when he was thirty-one. My Aunt Mary had lost my cousin Sammy when he was twenty-four, and my Aunt Miriam had married my Uncle Samir after his first wife, Heyam, passed away at age twenty-seven.

"I don't need you," I said.

The three women stood there looking sad for a moment longer. Then they vanished.

At the same moment, a scarlet man appeared before me. His skin was fire engine red. His shirt, pants, and shoes were red. Even his beard and the hair on his head beneath his cap were vividly red.

I knew who he was.

"Go away!" I shouted.

He laughed and began to dance around me.

"He's mine!" I screamed. "You can't have him! Go away! He is *mine*!"

A steady banging sound woke me with a start. Tommy was hammering on the wall between our rooms.

I jumped up and ran to his room. He looked at me. "Call 911."

I rushed back to my bedroom. As I dialed the phone I noticed the time on my clock radio: 12:45. I gave the 911 operator the necessary information, then ran to the front door and unlocked it. I also opened the garage doors. I wanted the responders to be able to get in easily.

Back at Tommy's side, I called the cardiology team and told the member on call what was going on. He said they'd be ready when we arrived.

It's strange, the things that go through your mind at times like that. As I've already said, denial is a powerful force.

I'll show you.

In my bedroom was a basket of unfolded laundry. I grabbed it and started to fold the clothes so they would be neat when the paramedics arrived. When I realized what I was doing, I stopped. But for those few moments, folding laundry meant that everything would be okay, that life would be normal.

Minutes later the paramedics swept in. As they were lifting Tommy onto the gurney, Nadia came home from an evening out with her friends—something she rarely did. She ran straight to her brother's side.

He looked at her and waggled his fingers. "I love you."

The paramedics placed him in the ambulance. When they offered me the option to ride in the back with them I said no, I'd drive myself. For one thing, I was sure Tommy would be fine; for another, that way I'd have a car to get home in later. For the same reasons, Nadia also drove separately.

Upon entering the hospital, she and I went to the check-in. Normally I was allowed to go straight to Tommy's beside, but this time the receptionist asked me to take a seat. "You can go back as soon as they get your son stabilized."

Nadia and I went to the waiting room. It was quarter to three in the morning. We sat next to each other, our heads bent and touching. The movie *Cocoon* was playing on the television.

One of the paramedics, a woman, walked through the waiting room on her way outside. Although I didn't pick up on it at that moment (denial), she seemed to be shaking her head ever so slightly (denial).

Next a doctor came out, sat down in front of me and asked me to tell him exactly what had happened that day. I recounted everything I could remember. When I asked how Tommy was, the doctor said, "We're still settling him." I remember thinking it was strange that settling him was taking so long (denial).

At 3:15 AM the same doctor came out, accompanied by one of Tommy's cardiologists, and asked Nadia and me to accompany them. We did as he asked, although something inside pulled at me not to go (denial).

We entered a small room just off the ER waiting room, and Nadia sat on one of the chairs. I stood in front of her.

The cardiologist was quiet and looked sad, but it was the doctor who spoke. "I'm sorry. We did everything we could."

Nadia let out a sob.

I didn't. I reached out, clutched the doctor by the lapels of his jacket and yelled (denial), "You fix him! You go back in there and *fix* him!"

Tears streamed down the cardiologist's cheeks. He took my hand. At his touch I collapsed into tears and growled in anguish. I grabbed my daughter, trying to comfort her and at the same time looking for her to comfort me. My baby was gone! *No!* My baby couldn't be gone, but he was! We clung to one another and sobbed.

And sobbed.

I don't know how long we stayed like that, but eventually the doctor told us they'd bring Tommy to a room where we could sit with him for a bit. They also gave us a telephone so we could contact whomever we needed to reach.

I went into the room. Tommy wasn't there yet. I called my brother, Anton, and asked him to phone our parents.

How do you tell people that your child, your baby, is dead? With each word you utter, you swear the lump in your throat will choke you.

Orderlies brought Tommy into the room, and Nadia and I looked at my son. Eighteen years old and so beautiful. He looked peaceful, serene. Nadia and I were amazed by the appearance of his skin. Before he passed, his arms had been bruised from all the failed attempts to draw blood from his collapsed veins. Now his skin was pristine, pure, as if he had never undergone any trauma.

Nadia and I looked at one another. At that moment I knew God had taken away the ugliness, the suffering, and the horrific pain Tommy had gone through for so many years, and replaced them with beauty.

My son was at peace.

She drives home with her daughter. They need to shower and change and get to her parents' house. There are funeral arrangements to make.

She realizes that for the first time in her life, even though she's facing utter tragedy, she feels no desire to eat.

She looks at the sky. The sun is starting to break through the clouds. Rain must have fallen at some point after they arrived at the emergency room, because suddenly a rainbow bends across the sky.

It has to mean that God has welcomed Tommy into heaven.

She'd swear she sees her son's face in a passing cloud.

STANDING NAKED
BEFORE YOU

Hundreds of people make their way through the room to pay their respects. She hears someone whisper that the line stretches out of the mortuary into the parking lot. Someone else says there are at least six hundred people in attendance.

She doesn't see any of them, really. She shakes hands, accepts kisses and condolences, but sees no one. No one except her son in his beautiful casket. She feels shattered, broken, irreparable.

The only thing she wants is to have her baby back. If she can't have that, she wants to lie in the casket next to him. She might as well; she feels dead inside.

Why are these people talking to her? Don't they know she can't hear them, doesn't really see them? Aren't they aware of the endless sea of hands washing over her, gripping her shoulder, of the tears running down their own cheeks as they observe the abject agony on her usually cheerful face?

These rituals are meant to pay respect, to send off the dead, to console the souls of those left behind, suffering, too numb to wish for the deaths they will crave once they begin to feel again.

For her they do not work.

The death of my son Tommy was, and at times still is, unbearable. For a while I prayed for death. I thought about killing myself, but I was afraid of what that would do to my daughter. We—my daughter and I—were all we had left. Steven and Nick were now both living in Florida.

For the next four months I barely slept or ate. My sister stayed with me, sleeping at the foot of my bed. My daughter couldn't sleep alone. Every night she lay down next to me. After she was asleep I would get up, go out and sit in the living room, and stare into space.

I buried Tommy on a Thursday and returned to work on Monday. I felt a responsibility to my job—and truth be told, I didn't know what else to do.

But tears were always close to the surface. The smallest display of heartache from my patients, or anyone asking me how I was doing, would send me into a tornado of sobbing; uncontrollable, agonizing cries of pain.

For the first time in my life, even food could not numb my desolation. I had no appetite. Ironically—and also for the first time in my life—my family kept encouraging me to eat something, anything.

The weight certainly came off. In six months I dropped from 413 pounds to 376. But even that was unimportant.

Nine months after the death of my son I still felt unbelievable desperation. While driving to and from work I fantasized about driving off a bridge.

Again, the only thing that kept me from doing anything so rash was my daughter. I couldn't put her through another death. We struggled to support one another. Although my poor Nadia needed my reinforcement, I was usually incapable of giving it to her. I tried to be strong, but the pain was so deep, so unimaginable.

One night as Nadia broke down crying she told me she had no one to turn to when she felt desolate over the loss of her brother.

"You have me," I said.

She shook her head. "No, Mom. Even when you try to help me, *I* end up supporting *you.*"

It wasn't until seven years later, after Nadia had her first child, that she told me she finally understood the volume of grief I must have felt. As much as she loved her brother, now that she had her own daughter she knew that nothing could compare to the love of a mother for her child.

I resented God for taking my son, and I resented life for giving me reasons and responsibilities for which to go on living.

When I realized my thoughts were turning dark more and more often, I went to see my physician. That was a huge moment for me. I realized that no matter how sad I was, I wasn't ready to die. I wanted to live.

But I needed help.

By that time Tommy had been dead for a year. When I stepped on the scale at the doctor's office I saw that the weight I had lost the first few months after Tommy's death was creeping back on.

My doctor put me on antidepressant medication. I had never taken antidepressants before. Even after I came home a basket case following my divorce, I'd fought my way back on my own. This time I didn't know what to do.

For three months I was on those antidepressants. Then I threw them away.

The epiphany came one day in late February. I don't know if my experience will make sense to you, but it was life-changing for me.

While dressing for work that morning I spent some time deciding whether to wear burgundy or brown. If you knew anything about me you'd know that I'm always very color-coordinated, that I love makeup, that I'm all about accessories matched to my outfits.

I made my choices and went to work. Three hours later I needed to use the ladies room. As I stood and pulled up my pants I realized I was wearing burgundy pants and *brown* shoes. Then, as I was washing my hands, I looked in the mirror and saw that for makeup I'd chosen tones of brown instead of burgundy.

That was when I knew the antidepressants were diminishing my mental capacities. Although I was no longer constantly sobbing, I was also not at my best even when it came to making simple decisions like matching my makeup to my clothing.

Although this revelation might sound silly and superficial, it was not. We all have certain things about us that are just part of what we are, habits that are as natural to us as breathing. This was one of mine.

Knowing that I wanted to go on living meant that I was feeling again—feeling fully. Although the pain was as fresh as it had been the day Tommy passed, I was no longer in shock, no longer numb. I had reached the point where I had to deal with the tumult within myself.

My old self-preservation habits returned in full force. I began to do what I've always done best to keep myself from hurting too deeply: I ate.

I ordered Applebee's Curbside, picked up my food, brought it home and gobbled it down. Sometimes, as I stuffed French fries and riblets down my throat, tears poured down my cheeks. I choked my tear-soaked French fries down anyway, as if to stuff down my pain. I hurt so badly...and as crazy as it sounds, food got me through.

I admit there were times when I consciously thought that if I ate enough maybe I would die. And that would be okay with me. Surely, dying from stuffing my body with high-calorie foods wasn't suicide. I was fat, and I'd just lost my son; no one would blame me for being depressed about his passing, would they? Everyone would understand why I gorged myself to death.

I know, it sounds horribly gruesome and depressing. But life seemed so unfair, so cruel. I just felt horribly, horribly cheated.

From my plate of Applebee's food I would contemplate my life. Despite what I'd believed when I saw Adam Taylor standing at the foot of the stairs at the convention, he had not been the man of my dreams. Our marriage had not been, as the Arabs say, "*Il nasee-b*"—"meant to be." I'm ashamed to admit that the day I asked Adam for the divorce, I had truly hoped he would say, "Linda, I love you. We have things to talk about; we'll work it out."

This was what he actually said: "You're crazy. We have four children."

So I felt cheated by my husband. Cheated by his indifference. I still felt like a failure for coming home a divorced mother of four, and without my eldest son.

Picking up the pieces had taken so long. Faking happiness on the outside when I felt devastation on the inside had been torturous. Pretending everything was going to be okay, and displaying the positive attitude I am so famous for, when all I wanted to do was to run far away, was destructive.

Then I lost Tommy, and that pushed me over the edge. Once again I tried to seem okay, but that time I failed. I no longer believed, as I once had, that everything would turn out fine. How could it? How *could* it when I hated the fact that I woke up still breathing every morning?

But not long after I flushed the anti-depression pills down the toilet, I began to realize I no longer felt that way. I had reached the point where instinctual survival kicked in. That, and the acceptance of things I could not change. I'd done everything I could to save my son, and I had failed. Although I didn't know why Tommy's time on earth had been cut so short, I decided I had to start fighting for my *own* life.

Eating myself into an early grave would, after all, have disappointed my son.

She looks at herself in the mirror and wonders what she weighs. Her bathroom scale only goes up to three hundred pounds. For years she'd gone to the Kaiser Positive Choice weight loss center to weigh herself whenever she wanted to face the truth and be accountable to what she was doing to her body. She'll do that again later today, after she calls her doctor and begs him to help her.

It's time to do something. She must lose weight.

At Kaiser she waits in line as one person after another weighs in prior to going to one of the classrooms designated for their program. Now it's her turn. She steps onto the scale and should have been shocked at the number that comes up on the printout: four hundred and thirty pounds.

No. She's not too surprised.

Her doctor's appointment is two days away. She wishes it was today.

BYPASSING MY PROBLEM

CHAPTER 9

The huge mound of spaghetti will soon be replaced by a second helping. She loves her spaghetti. Heck, she loves all things pasta. She should have been born Italian. Hey, maybe she *was* Italian in another life.

She has the house to herself tonight. Her daughter is at work. Old movies play on the television set; Fred Astaire and Ginger Rogers dominate the screen. Her favorites. She has the whole night to eat all she wants and to watch old musicals. She loves to pretend she's Ginger Rogers.

She laughs out loud at herself. Imagine Fred Astaire trying to do lifts with her throughout a dance move! She laughs harder, thinking that if he dropped her and she landed on him, no one would ever even see him under her.

That's funny, she thinks.

A perfect night at home. Old movies and a huge plate of spaghetti. Doesn't get much better than that.

In the spring of 2005 I went back to my doctor and told him I had thrown away the antidepressants.

"I want to lose weight," I said. "I want to do gastric bypass."

He had known and cared for me for years.

"No," he said.

"But—"

"Too many patients have died after having gastric bypass surgery. I'm not about to add you to the list of fatalities, Linda."

He suggested that I look into the wellness center at Kaiser because they offered many types of programs for weight loss. He even suggested Optifast, but I reminded him that I'd tried that program ten years earlier and had lost over ninety pounds in three months, only to gain it all back.

I left his office disheartened, feeling doomed to be fat. I didn't know what to do next. All I could think of was that I wanted to lose weight, and I needed help.

My mother's words rang in my ears: "Linda, you always accomplish everything you set out to do. Why do you have such a time controlling your weight?"

I always quipped, "Hey, Mom, I can't be perfect at *everything*. Only one man was ever perfect."

But her question was valid. Why was losing weight and keeping it off such a hurdle for me? What was holding me back, other than myself? The answer was obvious: nothing.

Nothing!

There is no reason to fail at weight loss. Of course there are lots of obstacles on the path to losing weight, but the bottom line is that we have to want to get thinner more than we want to self-medicate with food; we have to want to lose weight *badly*.

It's necessary for us to get it into our skulls that binge eating will never solve our problems, never correct our failures, never make us feel better in the long term. Binge eating does not replace lovers lost, loved ones who have died; it doesn't mitigate hardships within our families, difficulties dealing with work or the loss of work. Bingeing only sickens our bodies and fogs our brains, tricking us into fleeting moments of unawareness that are soon replaced with negativity, guilt, and dissatisfaction with ourselves and our lives.

I know this now, but at the time I couldn't see it. I was too lost in grief to recognize the damage I was doing to myself. Frankly, I did care about my rising weight— just not enough to do anything about it.

Part of me was secretly glad the doctor had said "no" to gastric bypass surgery. While frightened by my weight, I was nevertheless scared about taking such drastic action. The doctor saying "no" gave me a built-in excuse to make the easier choice.

Another year passed. Nadia and I helped each other get through the difficult times when one of us succumbed to grief. Bit by bit we began to laugh again. We had always been close; now we were all one another had.

But by February of 2006 I could no longer stand myself. I had to get that excess weight off. For the first time in my life, I felt every single pound I carried around with me.

So I made another appointment with my doctor. There had to be some kind of appetite suppressant available, or something else he could do to help me.

You won't believe what happened. He checked me over, did some lab work, and then sat me down in his office and looked me in the eye.

"Linda, I think you should have gastric bypass surgery."

I gaped. "Last year you told me not to. You told me about all the fatalities. What's changed that you'd recommend it now?"

"Kaiser researched why so many surgeries were failing. Turns out it was a lack of education; patients didn't know how to care for themselves properly *after* surgery. But now Kaiser has a 24-week education class to teach patients about their aftercare. It's been immensely successful."

That was all I had to hear. I went home, called the wellness center, and signed up for the next class.

The classes were led by professional counselors whose primary job was to drill into us the good, the bad, and the ugly facts of gastric bypass surgery. Nothing was held back, including the fact that one of the requirements was that we had to lose ten percent of our current weight before the surgeons would even consider us as candidates for surgery. At the time, the reason for this requirement—which is no longer used—was to help us de-fat our livers.

Over the first twelve weeks I lost only eight pounds, but by week thirteen something like a switch went off in my brain. Suddenly I really *believed* in my decision to have surgery. I felt that I was ready to change my life.

By week 24 I had lost over forty-seven pounds: four more than my ten-percent target.

I was in.

My surgery went well. For four or five days afterward I felt sore, but I never needed to open the bottle of liquid painkiller, Tylenol 3, I'd been given. Other than pure exhaustion, I felt pretty good.

Ironically, during the month I was off work I became addicted to the Food Network channel. I watched it practically from sunup to sundown, copying down the recipes I planned to make for everyone else.

Nadia teased me. "You just had surgery to lose weight, and all you think about is cooking."

Crazy, huh?

As soon as possible I returned to work. At the end of each day I'd come home and cook fabulous meals from the recipes I had garnered from the Food Network. My family and friends loved those meals, and were astounded at how I could cook them and not eat them.

"It's easy," I said. "I can't hold down very much food myself."

I had the surgery in October, and by February I had lost 110 pounds. Within a year I'd lost an additional 138 pounds.

My weight was down to 185 pounds, and I felt sensational! My surgeon, Dr. Tanaka, called me his poster child; I was doing everything right.

When I expressed concern about all the loose skin on my body he told me I was now carrying around 20 to 25 pounds of skin that would have to be surgically removed. In my head, all I could think about was this: if I didn't have all that excess skin my weight would be 160, not 185! What a freak I am.

But what I told the doctor was, "First I want to lose another twenty-five to thirty pounds."

He looked doubtful. "You probably won't lose much more weight. What's most important is that your lab tests show you're a very healthy woman now."

It was true. I was no longer diabetic. I no longer had high blood pressure. I could throw away the countless medications I'd been taking for those ailments.

A monumental sense of peace fell over me. For the first time since I was a young girl, I was *healthy*. At the age of forty-nine I had eradicated all the damage I'd caused my body. Gastric bypass surgery had saved my life.

I left Tanaka's office and called my parents to give them the great news. As I drove to work I said a prayer thanking God for giving me this second chance at health, for giving me back my life—and most of all for giving me something to look forward to for the first time since Tommy's death.

I vowed I would never take this gift from God for granted. He'd given medical scientists the ability to find this solution to help people like me lose weight; now it was up to me to keep that weight off.

Up to me...

She stands before the bathroom mirror after stepping off the scale. She loves her new body. It will never be like it was in her late teens, but she doesn't care. She looks slender. She looks normal. No one can see the loose skin beneath her clothes.

Even if she never has the money to have all that skin removed, she doesn't care. She feels so good in her body, excess skin and all. She can move again! She has amazing energy! Far more than she had before.

Energy is her life source. There's so much she wants to do. So much in the world she wants to experience. Nothing is going to stop her now. Certainly not a plate of spaghetti. Certainly not a chocolate bar.

Nothing.

THE COMEBACK KID

CHAPTER 10

As she's opening the door of the convenience store, a young, handsome man jumps forward to do it for her. He purposely holds the door in such a way that she has to brush against him as she passes. She gives him a brilliant smile. A look of appreciation comes over his face, and he smiles back.

She's noticed that since she's lost weight again, men open doors for her readily, and stare at her as they drive past, and constantly hit on her. Not since she was in her late teens and early twenties has she received so much attention from men. It surprises her.

Her friends and family tease her because she's usually clueless when men hit on her. Why wouldn't she be, having led such a sheltered life prior to her marriage, and having not dated in the nineteen years afterward? She's still quite naïve.

On the other hand, for the first time since her divorce she feels good enough about herself to really want to *meet and date someone. Is it too late for her? Can she possibly find someone who will love her in the way she needs to be loved?*

Even now, she doesn't care about looks as much as character. The man she chooses has to be a good person, decent, responsible and hard-working.

She laughs at the last characteristic. What if she meets a retired man? At her age, it's possible. She's never thought about that before....

With my new levels of energy I felt like there was nothing I couldn't do. I felt light and graceful. I felt beautiful.

Every night after work I went to the YMCA, took water aerobics for an hour, then went into the work-out room and used weights before finishing up with a thirty to forty-five minute run on the treadmill.

For the first time since my early twenties my rib bones showed, and my collarbones stuck out in feminine curves. My neck was long and grace-ful, my wrists small and dainty. My eyes appeared even larger in my face. And I had hipbones again! Even with the excess skin hanging around my hips, I could feel my hipbones protruding! Best of all, I could even cross my legs.

When the Y offered aerobics or Jazzercise classes, I took them. I even joined a hip-hop class because I wanted to learn how to dance that way. Apart from one other brave old woman, the other participants were teenagers. Still, I'm proud to say I held my own in that class.

I became ever more adventurous. My friend Janice, a gastric bypass class buddy, took classes with me. We learned ballroom dancing and salsa. Janice is also a hiker who especially loves walking up mountains. She asked me if I wanted to hike up Iron Mountain—a seven-mile round trip. I said I would.

This would be a whole new challenge for me. Seven miles up and down a mountain? I had never done anything like that before.

We met at six a.m. and drove to the entrance of the trail. It was a beautiful morning, a bit overcast and cool, but the day promised to become warm and spectacularly sunny.

As we traversed the trail up the mountainside, I told Janice all about my recent first date with a guy named Chris. She wanted every detail.

I told her he'd offered to take me to dinner but I wasn't sure I wanted to spend that kind of time with him, so I suggested we get a frozen yogurt in the afternoon. That way, we'd have an opportunity to talk and get to know one another without the pressure of a long meal in front of us. He loved the idea.

We met and enjoyed a frozen yogurt. I learned a great deal about him. He loved music, especially country music. He had a 21 year old son with a drug problem. Due to financial difficulties he and his ex-wife still lived together, even though they had been divorced for years. Also, he smoked pot.

In his truck we listened to some of his favorite music, and he tried to talk me into taking him back to my place and having sex. I said no. In fact, I told him I wouldn't be seeing him again.

"I don't date guys who do drugs, or who have ex-wives living with them," I said. He looked upset, but said he understood.

Chris was nice, but throughout our conversation, I got the impression he was looking for someone to move in with and help pay for his lifestyle and have sex with him. That was pretty much all of it.

I chalked the whole thing up to experience. I figured I'd trust my instincts. Just because a man was humorous and charming didn't mean he was a potential mate. Besides, I wasn't sure I wanted any type of permanent relationship with anyone.

Janice shared with me the attention she was also getting these days. It was fun discussing men with her. All this interest from men just because we were thinner!

Thinking back, I'm not sure what was easier to accomplish: hiking to the top of a mountain, or dealing with attention from men. But I will tell you this: when I reached the summit of Iron Mountain that day, I felt wonderfully proud of myself. I'd just done something I had never done before. The accomplishment was exhilarating. Even when I slipped and slid on my ass for ten feet down the mountainside, I still felt incredible. Who would have thought that this once-upon-a-time fat woman would ever lose enough weight or gain enough strength and stamina to climb a mountain?

But navigating the dating world was a whole different experience of unfamiliarity. Don't get me wrong. I loved (and still love) the attention. Flirting is so much fun—but for me, to take that forward into a more intimate relationship was a terrifying concept.

I kept thinking that with my luck, I'd give myself up to some man only to find out two weeks later that I'd contracted a disease. What would I say to my children and family then?

You're probably asking yourself, "Is this woman for real?" Yes, I am. Basically, I considered myself a born again virgin. Don't laugh...although even I have to admit it's both funny and pathetic. There I was, a grown woman who had borne four children and was now a grandmother, scared about having sex with a man.

I just wasn't sure it would be worth it. And to be honest, I didn't expect to meet anyone I could get serious with anyway. Because of my upbringing, my standards were high, although not any higher than what I demanded of myself. Integrity and character were very important to me.

One night I went dancing with two of my girlfriends, Amanda and Janice, at a dive steak house bar that featured karaoke several nights a week. The steaks were decent there, and the karaoke nights catered to people close to my age.

It was a fun, laid-back kind of place where everyone got to know everyone else. It reminded me of the television series *Cheers*. People were friendly without applying any pressure.

Amanda, Janice, and I could not sing. Dance, yes... well, except for Janice. She had no rhythm, but still, she got out there and had fun. As for me, I'd made up my mind that I was going to apply my general "it will all work out" life's philosophy to meeting a man: "Have fun. Don't go looking for someone. Just enjoy yourself. If someone is attracted and interested, he'll make a move, and we will see how it goes. If no one shows an interest, at least you had a good time with your friends."

At that bar I did meet one man who was really cute. He owned his own business, and every week he took his employees out for a fun night at this particular karaoke bar. He challenged me to get up there and sing. No way! But I told him if *he* got up and sang, my friend and I would be his personal go-go dancers.

He sang his heart out while I did my best gyrating dance moves. It was pretty hot.

Losing weight had created opportunities. I went out on several first dates, and always left as friends. All the guys were very nice, but by the end of our time together it was easy to see they weren't looking for the same things in life as I was.

My closest friends told me that my expectations were too high. So I relaxed a bit, and met even more nice people. Everyone I went out with, even if only once, remained on friendly terms with me. Still, I knew we were not going to go anywhere as far as a relationship was concerned.

I'll admit there was another reason I was leery about undressing in front of a man: although I loved my sexy new body, it was still wrapped in all that excess skin. As long as I had clothes on, nobody could really see that.

Clothing made all the difference. I loved shopping for new clothes, especially since I now had all the mall shops at my disposal, whereas previously my only real choices had been Lane Bryant and Catherine's.

Heels! Beautiful sexy heels! Now I had a much greater selection of shoes to choose from. It was wonderful.

The only heels I avoided were six-inch stilettos; there was no way I could wear them without falling on my ass. But I did try them on. Sexy! Sexy!

My life was wonderful. Even though I did have one serious problem in my life (sorry, not ready to talk about that yet), the fact that I felt so good about myself ensured that I could handle any problem better than I would have before.

Or so I thought. The future would prove differently.

On the medical front, every doctor's appointment went perfectly. My blood work results were ideal. My physician was thrilled with my success. In fact, I gave lectures to other gastric bypass patients at Kaiser. I loved talking to the people attending the same twenty-four week class I had taken. I reinforced to them one point my counselor, Nancy, had impressed upon our group: gastric bypass is only a tool. If after the procedure is over you do not take care of yourself properly, you can gain the weight back.

I made clear to my classes that such regained weight is not the result of an over-nourished body. Bypass patients do not absorb nutrients, only calories; post-surgery weight gain is like malnourishment in reverse.

The best part of giving the lectures was the response I received from the wonderful people who attended. They told me I inspired them and gave them the hope of living the kind of life everyone wants so desperately. On top of that, lecturing others helped me keep myself on track.

So did the overall health improvements I enjoyed. For those in my group, the surgery rid us of diabetes and high blood pressure. Others who had required constant oxygen or could no longer get around without the aid of a walker or electric chair were now off oxygen and could walk on their own accord.

As I said, gastric bypass surgery saved my life. It changed me, and not only physically—it changed my entire life. My surgeon headed the surgical group at Scripps Mercy hospital, with which Kaiser contracted to perform bypass surgeries. This group's success ratings were much higher than the national averages. I felt truly blessed to have been given this chance.

Had I not persisted in my desperate fixation on losing weight, I'm not sure I would be alive today. The classes developed by Kaiser and Scripps Mercy provided the tools needed to do well after surgery. They also forced me to take a hard look at myself. For example, I learned just how bad I was at setting boundaries. I have always had—and still have—a difficult time saying "no" to people, even when I should. This flaw had cost me a great deal in the past, and soon would again.

You see, I was brought up to always do the right thing; I hate disappointing anyone. So although I've always been a tigress when it comes to sticking up for others, I'm horrible at standing up for myself.

Ironically, I taught my children that "If you're right-handed you cannot cut off your right hand," meaning that you cannot give your last dime to help someone else if you need that dime just as desperately. But it turns out that when it comes to making things happen for other people, I myself *am* willing to cut off my right hand (and yes, I'm right-handed).

In the Kaiser classes I learned that saying "no" to someone is not a bad thing. We were adults who shouldn't have to ask anyone else to resolve our issues. Telling other people "yes" in situations in which we were accepting responsibility for them not only burdened us, it stunted their personal growth, preventing them from accessing the tools needed to solve their own problems. Instead, they would continue to make the same mistakes over and over—and continue to call upon us to bail them out.

On the other hand, telling those people "no" because it's the right thing to do for us empowers us to no longer allow others to take advantage of us or make us responsible for their carelessness.

When we don't set boundaries for others, it's the equivalent of not putting our own needs first. This resonated with me. As life kept telling me—and I kept ignoring—when you don't put your own needs first, you're bound to allow negative issues to interfere with the life you deserve and the person you're meant to be.

Denying yourself respect is a recipe for failure, frustration, depression, and anger. These feelings, in turn, lead us to revert to the old habits we've worked so hard to overcome: in my case, binge eating.

As you can see, these classes were very beneficial. I made friends from my class that I still keep in touch with to this day; we even formed our own support group that met weekly for several years.

Then there were the conventions.

The surgeons at Scripps Mercy generously created an annual convention for their gastric bypass patients. It was a two-day event that brought together people from all around the world who had been patients of this surgical team.

It was held at a local hotel. The first night, Friday, was the time for people to meet and share their experiences, followed by a talent show.

On Saturday many of us would meet very early in the morning for a walk around the community led by one of the surgeons. Upon our return, breakfast was served.

Now I have to share this with you. The hotel in which the convention was held is very good, known for its many amenities, its service, and particularly its cuisine....

...Except when it came to food for gastric bypass patients. *Ugg! Ick! Eyew!* Our breakfast consisted of dry scrambled eggs, fruit salad and tortillas. Although fruit salad was a fine choice, most of us patients could not keep down tortillas. And did I mention the scrambled eggs were very dry? *Ick!*

But that's all right because food wasn't so important to us anymore, right?

Wrong! We were recovering food addicts, so of course food was important to us—especially because we could eat so little of it.

But we soldiered on. For the rest of Saturday, classes were offered on many well- thought-out subjects—plastic surgery to get rid of the loose skin; or, for women, breast lifts so those parts no longer dragged on the floor. There were nutrition classes and motivational/life coaching classes, among many other offerings. I learned a great deal about caring for myself.

Best of all, I was inspired and motivated by other people's stories of how their lives had been changed for the better by their surgery, or how their family members were finally relieved from worry and stress.

In the evening the classrooms in the hotel magically merged into a single large ballroom for dinner and dancing, following a fashion show. Again, I don't know what the chefs at this hotel were told about our needs, but most of the food was inedible. Chicken breast—dry; flavorless mashed potatoes; salad (that was good); blanched green beans and dinner rolls followed by Jell-O and tapioca goblets for dessert: every year, that was the convention's menu.

Unfortunately gastric bypass patients cannot eat dry or blanched foods, especially within the first two to three years of their surgery, because we cannot digest them. If we try to do so we end up in the bathroom vomiting. I solved this problem by eating only the salad.

I'm proud to share with you that for two years I was in the convention's fashion show. What was best about that was that it meant you got up on the catwalk and strutted your new, sexy body as a huge movie screen showed a "before" picture and bio of you. It was cool to see how far people had come after having gastric bypass surgery—their evolution into healthy, active, energetic people fulfilling their personal goals.

The third convention I attended had a Hawaiian theme. Again I modeled, and this time chose the music I wanted played as I strutted my stuff on the runway. I picked Shakira's "Hips Don't Lie." I thought it was fitting—plus, when I reached the end of the runway, I paused and did some serious belly dancing. From the audience came whoops and hollers. I felt fearless!

That same terrible dinner was served after the show. I picked at my salad. I'd come alone that year because my friends from my gastric bypass group had not signed up in time. After dinner the DJ got busy playing dance hits from many different genres. That was all I needed: once I heard the beat, I had to get out on the dance floor, shut out the world and move to the music.

I asked the ladies I'd met at my table to get up and join me. Soon we were all out there, working up a sweat, dancing to song after song. I hadn't felt so good about my body and myself since I was in my mid to late teens.

While I was on the dance floor a man approached me, a look of blatant desire in his intense green eyes. He introduced himself as Bob and asked me to dance. We did so—including a very nice slow dance.

I liked the way this man held me. I loved the way he looked at me. I noticed that we fit together perfectly as we swayed to the music. Being in this stranger's arms felt comfortable, yet passionate and intense— an embraceable need fulfilled.

After a few more dances my new acquaintance showed me his "before" photo. He'd lost two hundred and seventeen pounds and looked amazing.

He asked me if I wanted to step out into the hallway and talk. I don't know why I said yes, except that he seemed really nice.

We made our way out of the ballroom and into a hallway where a tiny, elegant bench was waiting. As we settled onto it I started to giggle.

"What's so funny?" he asked.

"Before our surgeries, this bench would have been a single seat for either one of us. Now we can both sit on it with room to spare."

He laughed, and we started talking—or I should say *he* started talking...and would not, could not, stop. His name was Bob Wagner. He told me everything, and I do mean everything, about his life. He put more out there about himself and his family and his past relationships than most people would to a person he or she hadn't known for at least six months.

But Bob spat it all out, as if failing to do so meant he might actually perish. Even when he asked me questions, I never got to finish answering before he took the conversation over again. He also kept rubbing his hands together as if he was washing them over and over again. I don't know why he was so nervous, but I thought it was adorable and kind of cute. Although he often didn't look at me as he went on and on, when he did raise his green eyes, his gaze was so intense I could tell he really cared what I thought about him.

Later he would tell people that he was testing me to see if I would run away—but after I got to know him, I realized that his need to spit out his entire life story was just the way he was. He told the same story to everyone, and I do mean *everyone*, he encountered— waitresses, family members, desk clerks. The habit was simultaneously annoying, charming, and honest.

It wasn't until the DJ was rolling her gear out of the ballroom that we noticed the time: one o'clock. In the morning. We had been sitting there talking for four hours. He had been talking, anyway. Fortunately I'm an incredible listener.

"One o'clock?" I said. "Oh, I have to go."

"Can I have your phone number? Can we email one another?"

I answered without hesitation: "Sure."

We made our way to the front desk, where he asked the clerk for pen and paper. We exchanged information and Bob offered to walk me to my car.

"Sure," I said, again without hesitation.

We left the hotel—and I don't know why I did this, but I took his hand in mine. We walked hand in hand toward my car. I felt safe with him. His hand felt so right in mine. It was as if they belonged together. I had a hard time letting go when we reached my car.

He opened the door for me. Before I could climb in he said, "May I kiss you?"

"Sure."

It was a great first kiss. His lips were soft and master-ful, gentle and sexy all at once. *Roooaaaaar!* When we pulled apart he looked at me, and I knew he wanted to ask me to stay. I also knew that he wouldn't ask.

Our evening had the makings of the start of some-thing special.

He placed his lei around my neck, and I got into my car. As I pulled away I looked in the review mirror and saw him standing in the parking garage watching me.

I hoped he would call me the next day.

As I drove home, and for the first time since divorc-ing Adam twenty-one years before, I felt a quiet inner excitement, like a small flame lighting a large dark room. I wondered: if Bob had asked me to stay and talk further into the night, would I have? The answer was probably "yes."

On the drive home all I could think about was how much I would have loved him to have invited me to drive down to my favorite beach spot in La Jolla. I wanted to sit with him watching the waves crash against the shore, the water lit by the moon and spar-kling with twinkling stars reflecting the night sky.

I smiled. Was it possible this man would change my life? I had to make an effort to not get over-excited. After all, despite his nonstop chatter I hardly knew him, and since my divorce I had met many very nice men. Still, there was one huge difference between Bob and those other men: none of the others had made me feel the way Bob did.

It was the expression in his eyes when he looked at me: a blend of a "man on a mission to possess the woman he desires" and "man nervous about the intensity of his feelings for a woman he barely knows."

I loved it.

Bob didn't give me much chance to decide if I liked him or not. The cliché "He swept me off my feet" is the only way I can express the railroading I got from this man who was so determined to love me and have my love in return.

The Saturday after the conference he came down to San Diego from Long Beach where he lived and worked, and we had an incredible day that ended with him cooking dinner for me. His feelings for me were obvious, overpowering, heady. I knew he wanted to stay with me, but I respected him more because he'd promised to take his daughter to Disneyland the next morning and had no intention of breaking his date with her.

Sunday morning came, and as I went about my day I couldn't keep from thinking about Bob. I wondered if I was on his mind as well.

I got the answer early that afternoon when the phone rang.

"I can't stop thinking about you," Bob said. "I wish I were there holding you in my arms right now." Then: "Linda, I have to tell you something, and if after I tell you, you never want to see me again, I'll understand."

My stomach dropped. What could he possibly tell me that might make me not want to see him again?

"Linda...I just got a call from my doctor. I have leukemia. I knew I had it when I met you, but my doctor just told me they'd misdiagnosed the type I have, and the chemo treatments I've already undergone aren't effective against the type of leukemia I have."

I realized I'd been holding my breath. Slowly, I let the air out of my lungs.

"What does this mean?" I said.

He started rattling off statistics and percentages regarding his chances of defeating his disease. He admitted that not only did he currently have leukemia, he had already suffered from three other forms of cancer, starting when he was nineteen. He had beat the disease every time, and was now determined to beat it yet again.

Then he added, "Linda, I'll understand if you don't want to see me anymore. I know what you went through with losing Tommy, and I don't want to put you through any more heartache."

I spoke firmly. "Bob, first of all, we barely know each other. Right now we're just friends getting acquainted. Second, I don't run away from my people just because they're sick. I run away from people if they're jerks. Your being sick does not mean we can't be friends and get to know one another."

I heard him release a long breath. "Before I met you all I wanted to do was die and have this over with. My only worry was about Jennifer being alone; I don't want her to lose another parent. But now...after meeting you and being with you, I want to live."

Then he added: "I never believed in love at first sight, but when I saw those eyes of yours across the dance floor, I started thinking about having a home with you, and what our life together would be like."

Funny, but those words scared me more than the ones about him having leukemia. Don't misunderstand: my heart went out to him and his daughter, who had lost her mother at three years of age and her stepmother six years later. For her to now have a father battling cancer must have been terrifying.

But Bob's declaration of love so soon after we met *terrified* me. How could he love me when he barely knew me? I was tempted to back away; his feelings seemed too intense too soon. I was frightened that if I let myself fall in love with him I could only get hurt. I had loved Adam even as I asked him for a divorce, but found that I couldn't go on living with a man who gave so little of himself. In fact he had once told me he didn't even believe in love—and gone on to prove it to me during the next twelve and three-quarter years.

In a single weekend Bob had already given me much, much more than that—which meant I also had more to lose.

But in the end, the bad news he gave me that Sunday did not frighten me away. As always, I looked for the sunlit side. Who knew what might develop between us? We might end up as only friends—but if something more was meant to be, well, who was I to deny it?

A scenario crossed my mind, and I described it to Bob: "What if we'd fallen in love and married, and then two years later, or ten years later, you got leukemia? Would I run away from you then? Of course not."

Which was why, despite my fears, I couldn't, wouldn't, and didn't break it off with him that Sunday.

Not everyone shared my feelings. When my mother, sister and brother heard about Bob's illness they were very concerned about me developing a relationship with him; they didn't want to see me go through another round of what I'd already suffered with Tommy. My friends were equally worried.

But in my heart I knew that I wasn't going to give up the chance of having a relationship with Bob simply because he was ill. Not only was there something about him that drew me, but what kind of a person would I be if I severed a relationship with anyone due to illness? That's not who I am.

There was another factor to consider as well. When I lost Tommy I lost my fear of death. I can't fear something that entered my soul and that I feel every day that I stand here on earth; death stayed behind along with the memories of my son. Even now, ten years later, the pain of his death often feels fresh, forcing me into an unwelcome but profound acceptance of mortality.

So I left the door of my heart open for Bob, not knowing that his entry into my life would prove to be more than just the beginning of a new chapter for me. It would soon challenge the relationships I had with all the other people I most love.

I was about to pay a heavy price for loving Bob.

Men her own age or older come with a different set of problems than young men. They might have health issues, or have been divorced one or more times; they could have children with one or more women. But there are also positive attributes to that age group: maturity, usually greater financial security, more confidence, and being prepared for a real relationship—assuming they aren't habitual "players," of course.

Speaking of that, what about sex? Oh my God! She's had only one partner in her entire life: her ex-husband. She wonders if she even knows what to do in bed anymore.

Then there are all the sexually transmitted diseases out there to worry about. How do you know if a potential partner has one? Do you just ask? Make them take a blood test? What?

And how soon should she agree to have sex? For her that's a huge question. She's forty-nine. Other women her age sleep with whomever they feel like, just because—but she wasn't raised that way. Should she wait until after a certain number of dates, or until she's engaged, or what?

And what do men expect, sexually, these days? She's confused and unsure of herself. Thank goodness she has great friends to advise her: smart, savvy more-than-first-generation American women, women no longer bound by strictures of the old country, who know a thing or two about sex, men, and modern expectations.

Wait...first she has to figure out what her OWN expectations are. What should count most now are her own feelings; she doesn't want to do something foolish and have regrets....

25 POUNDS OF LOOSE SKIN

CHAPTER 11

He takes her into his arms. She's trembling, but as he presses her against him she can feel his desire for her growing. His lips find hers. She feels the need in him, but it only makes her feel even more uneasy.

His kisses are passionate, irresistible. Her body turns to hot melted butter as his lips find the spot beneath her earlobe. She sags against him.

As he begins to undress her she stiffens just a bit. He must have felt it too, for his hands stop their work while his lips plunder her mouth, not allowing her to think of anything except his desire.

She has not been with a man in this way since her divorce over twenty years before. And with Adam she had never experienced this type of passion: overwhelming, intoxicating, terrifying, sensual. This man fills her senses, clouding them to the point of blindness.

But shyness overtakes her as he finally stands naked before her, proud and knowing—knowing that before tonight she has been with only one other man in her life.

He seems to understand that there is only one way to overcome her nerves. Boldly, he reaches out and undresses her, at the same time kissing her lips, the spot below her earlobes, the base of her throat. Not letting her think clearly enough to pull away....

Instead he grows even more passionate and the fervor of his lovemaking overtakes her. She begins to give back to him, matching his movements in a sensual rumba.

That afternoon he makes love to her over and over again until neither of them can dance the dance any longer. Then he cradles her in his arms and they fall into a slumber of sweet satiation.

She is his...now, and forever.

I was terrified the first time Bob and I made love. I cannot tell you which was scarier; making love to a man I was just getting to know, or being naked in front of *any* man with all that loose skin still draping my body.

When I was lying on my back I didn't look so bad; my ribs stuck out and my legs looked muscularly slender and shapely—well, except for the "front butt."

For those of you who do not know what front butt is, let me explain. You know the very fatty loose skin at the top of your inner thighs that forms the shape of a small butt when you put your legs together? That's front butt. It's the result of excess skin not sagging fully after you lose a great deal of weight. Instead it stays rounded, forming a fleshy, fatty butt—but in front of your legs, right where the V forms.

If you lie down and bend your knees, you might be able to hide front butt between your thighs. That's the kind of thing you think about when you're fat or are equipped with extra skin after having been fat: how can I look less heavy; how can I disguise or cover up all this loose skin? Fat people learn all kinds of tricks to hide the not-so-pretty areas of our bodies. Why do you think Spanx were invented?

You know what I'm talking about. Even my thin friends have tricks that make them look more attractive, especially when their clothes are off. For example, when one of my girlfriends lies down, her large breasts hang toward her sides, leaving between them an open path like a landing strip where normally she would display beautiful cleavage. Her trick for giving herself cleavage while lying on her back is to fold her arms over her ribs and lift her breasts with them. I tried it; it works.

Given all this, I was terribly nervous about having sex with Bob. I thought I looked pretty good in clothes, but once the clothes came off all I could say about myself was, "Oh my God!" In addition to front butt, I had bat-wing underarms and an apron of loose skin stretching from one hipbone to the other.

Men are luckier, maybe because their bellies never have to stretch out from childbirth. When Bob stood before me naked, he was beautifully shaped and muscular, only a bit of loose skin hanging from his belly.

Life is sometimes not fair to women.

It was quite the shocker to me to have lost so much weight and still not have the body I truly wanted. Realistically, while I knew that I would never regain the body I'd had when I was eighteen, and that I'd have some loose skin—I hadn't imagined having *this much* of it. Up until I met Bob I'd been so grateful to have all the other weight off my body that I hadn't cared much about any of this. I'd never planned on getting married or expected to be naked in front of a man again. For me, dancing, flirting and occasionally making out with a man already comprised a huge step. Going further than that? Getting *naked*? Well, let's just say I only flirted with the idea.

Then there were the STDs. You have to remember that I married Adam in 1978. Three years later, AIDs and HIV were all over the news.

Fast-forward to 2007 and after. I was nervous about being physically intimate with a man even though I didn't know much about the kind of damage STDs could do to you, or for that matter what the differences were between one STD and another. Remember, I'd been raised in very sheltered circumstances.

Bob changed all that. For starters, he made me feel beautiful. He thought my body was beautiful.

"You're just hard up," I told him.

He laughed and said he had never been hard up.

"Then you must be blind," I said.

"I've never been blind, either," he replied.

Bob and I met on October 2, 2009.
He professed his love for me on October 11.
On December 5 he asked me to marry him.
I said "Yes."

I was deeply and irreversibly in love. Bob made me feel wanted and desirable, and promised that would never change. I would always feel loved, wanted, and needed. I believed him.

Four and a half years later, he's kept all his promises.

Sex with this man was and is passionate and fulfilling, fun and bawdy—and allows me to be myself completely. I am quite goofy and funny and sexual, and so is Bob.

Still, at times I get lost in deep thought. Most people never guess when my mind is far away worrying about things, but Bob always knows, and when he sees I'm lost in my world of worry he finds ways to make me smile. He appreciates and accepts me for who I am and understands what I am about. He makes me laugh. He makes me happy. He sees me as an amazing woman.

So here's the question: If I'm so happy and deeply in love, if I'm married to a man who says I'm the most beautiful woman he has ever seen (I'd hate to see what the other women in his life looked like!), how come I've gained back 115 of the 250 pounds I lost with my gastric bypass surgery?

So many things are changing all at once. Bob drives down from L.A. every Friday night and spends the weekend with her. Her daughter has moved out, gotten married, and is expecting a baby.

She should be completely happy, but there's a problem: all her children are at odds about her relationship with Bob. They are watching the relationship closely. They are unsure if Bob is right for her.

Although she feels immense pressure coming at her from all directions, she convinces herself she's successfully managing to juggle all the different balls of her life.

Denial. Her life is actually spiraling out of control. Too many of the people she loves and who love her are making her feel as if they are judging her every move.

Her descent begins with a handful of jellybeans. Just a small handful of jellybeans is all. How bad could that be?

Very, very bad: bad enough to ignite an atomic bomb. The damage unleashed by the explosion is her addiction to sugar. Once set free, her dormant desire to eat rises like a phoenix. Its powerful spell on her mind takes over everything she has accomplished in the last five years.

First a pound or two, then ten pounds gained. Her body is back to craving the poison that in the past led her into the insanity of food addiction and binge eating.

She tries to reign the monster in, to regain control, to right the ship of her life before it's too late.

But it's already too late.

PISSED

CHAPTER 12

*O*range, purple, and pink hues streak the deepening blue sky as the sun begins to set. As she sits staring into the distance, a peaceful feeling strums her heartstrings as sweetly as the breeze whispers across her bare arms. The vastness of the ocean always reminds her of how small she is in this world.

Yet her problems loom very large; whenever she thinks about them she feels as if she's drowning. If she walks into the ocean and REALLY drowns, will her inner pain finally go away? Or will it follow her into the afterworld?

This thought brings her back to reality: she can't escape either her problems OR her pain.

I'm angry. Why didn't I realize it before? Why didn't I notice how much rage I carry within me? It's like the fury I felt at God and life when Tommy was dying. After that, how could I not recognize my anger? How long have I been dragging it around?

Most importantly, have I been insane to not allow myself to experience this anger, address it, express it? No. The problem is not insanity. The problem stems from a childhood of downloading into my brain the message that I am not *allowed* to feel anger. It's not that anyone actually told me that; it's that I denied *myself* the right to get mad in order to avoid the kind of responses I got when I surrendered to rage.

As a result, to this day I cannot stay mad. Ever. Not even when I have a perfectly good reason to be furious; I simply cannot sustain it.

Why is that? Now, as I look back, the answer seems crystal clear: nice girls do what they are told. They never talk back; they always behave themselves. They are nice. They act like young ladies. It is unladylike to show anger, so shame on you if you act out!

That's what I believed was expected of me.

The truth is, all the hard work I'd applied to losing 250 pounds was not undone by a single bad weekend or even a single handful of jelly beans. It was undone by a lifetime spent denying things that should have made me very, very angry. I never allowed myself to feel my fury, to own it, and then to address it. Instead, I was patient and understanding. I was caring and loving. I was a *good girl*.

Ironically, I'm great at getting angry on behalf of other people. That kind of anger is acceptable because I only employ it when I feel that my children, other family members, or friends are being treated unfairly. I hate seeing anyone take advantage of others in general, but especially when the victims are people I know and care for.

But I never gave myself the same support. I stifled my feelings, literally stuffed them down inside me. If I showed the world only patience and understanding, I thought, if I placed other people's feelings above my own, that would make me special. It would make me the bigger person, so to speak. It would put me in control of the situation.

Now, if you were to mention this to my kids, they'd laugh. "My mom can get *really* mad," they'd say. "Trust me, I've felt her wrath!"

That's true. When it comes to my children and what I think is best for them, all I can say is, get the heck out of my way. Whether it's something they're doing or a situation I don't think is right, I will do whatever is necessary to convince them of what is in their best interests.

But that's not the kind of anger I'm talking about; that's the kind of anger a mother reveals when she's trying to protect and raise her children.

In my life there have been times when people I love have hurt me immeasurably. Yet even when my first husband chose not to do right by our children and me, I never got angry with him – not *consciously* angry. I felt sorry for him for letting go of me—a woman who would have loved, respected and cared for him till our dying days. I felt sad that he wasn't man enough to be a good father to his children, to spend time with them or try to be a part of their lives. I felt sorry for him because he did not value what he was missing, and basically threw us all away.

I was sad for him, and sad for my children, torn apart by the never-ending pain of the woulda-shoulda-coulda beens. Even after all these years a part of me still wondered: if my marriage to Adam had worked, would Tommy still be alive? I know that makes no sense, yet it seems that many of the problems in my life are directly related to my ex-husband. Certainly my eldest son Steven wouldn't have gone through all the hardships he suffered, including having a stepmother who could be cruel to him, if I hadn't divorced his father.

As for Nick . . . I knew how painful my divorce had been for him. He wanted his family to be together. He missed his father and his big brother. Yet the three years and nine months he eventually spent with his father and stepmother were awful for him. I don't think he ever completely got over the experience.

It was Nadia, my precious princess, who suffered the most. Even now her relationship with her father remains very tenuous. For some reason Adam was never there for her at all. Yet she is a remarkable young woman; if it weren't for her I don't know how I would have gotten through my life thus far. She was strength when I needed strength. She was humor when I needed to laugh. She was a shoulder when I needed to weep. She was a friend and confidante when I felt I could not express my truth to anyone else. She was wisdom when I did not want to see.

Still...even now I can't help thinking that if her father and I had made a success of our marriage, Nadia wouldn't have picked up my bad eating habits—or made other choices that increased the difficulty of her life. Of course, I realize that's just the way things are; in the real world people cannot always work their problems out. But children don't understand that some things just happen. Even if they're aware that "divorce" exists, they don't comprehend that it is something that can pull your family apart.

But I knew, and I knew there was no point in getting all angry about it.

I had convinced myself that Adam was an honorable man, but he wasn't. Nor was his family. Honorable people do not abandon their grandchildren and daughter-in-law when they know their son is doing them wrong. They don't stand aside when they see their son playing golf while his wife can't find the money to buy groceries or sanitary napkins.

I remembered a time when I was visiting my in-laws and mentioned that our house was about to be taken away due to foreclosure. I asked my father-in-law if my kids and I could move in with them until I figured out how I was going to support us and find a place to live. He refused. He said that his daughter "would not like having kids running around the house." In other words, it was more important to him that his daughter, Sarah, have a nice, quiet home than that his grandchildren and I not end up living on the streets.

Yet I didn't express any anger about it. Astonishment, maybe, but not anger.

I just didn't get it.

That's what put the weight back on me: suppressing my most valid emotions.

Psychologists suggest that when someone close to us dies we go through several emotional stages. In fact we *need* to go through these stages in order to move forward in life. Anger, they say, is the most critical stage of all. Well, I never got there, either when my marriage died or when my son died—and without acknowledging and expressing anger, we cannot release our pain.

When Bob asked me to marry him, I already knew that my children were not on board with the idea. My sons had never even met Bob, but my daughter, who *had* met him, did not like him—and had made her views known to her brothers.

I needed, like I need to breathe, for my children to share my happiness with me, so I tried to plan a wedding around their schedules. First I set July 2010 for the wedding date. But Steven said he couldn't leave his business then, and Nick's wife was due to have her baby. I understood.

Meanwhile I hoped Bob and I could take a trip to Florida to meet the boys, but that proved impossible as well. My father was ill, and Bob and I were both too busy to take off from work.

So, to poor Bob's frustration, I postponed the wedding. I absolutely had to find a date that would work for us but would also allow my children to be there.

But the holidays came and went and still my children were unavailable. It was a very busy time for Steven's business, and Nick was not interested in taking both a newborn baby and a one-year-old on a cross-country airplane flight.

So I realized if I wanted my children at my wedding, *we* would have to go to *them*. The next available date that would give both Bob and me enough time off was Memorial Day weekend.

I called my boys and told them Bob and I would come to Pensacola and get married there. The boys seemed excited.

Once again the planning process began. This time, instead of the big wedding I had originally intended to have in San Diego for friends and family, we would have a small wedding, just twenty of us, in Pensacola. My daughter and her husband Sean agreed to fly out for the ceremony with their daughter, Lenah. Bob's daughter, Jennifer, would join us as well.

At last, Bob and I would be married, blissfully surrounded by most of our children! I cannot tell you how excited I was.

I found a lovely family restaurant situated on a deck overlooking the Gulf of Mexico. It served baskets of fresh Gulf seafood, and would provide an arbor for us to marry under. There was an area for dancing with a live band that would play the evening of our wedding.

My daughter-in-law's best friend, Carrie, was an amateur photographer, and agreed to take pictures. I found a florist who would put together my bouquet, provide us with a ring bearer's pillow, and make a boutonniere for Bob. A bakery suggested by my daughter-in-law created a cake covered with handmade white chocolate seashells.

Everything was planned to the last detail. I bought a lovely wedding gown and gorgeous shoes from Nordstrom with a lace bolero beaded jacket and a veil from David's Bridal. At Macy's I found the right jewelry. When Bob and I boarded the plane to fly to Pensacola, I was as ready for the big day as any bride could ever be.

My excitement was matched by Bob's nervousness about meeting my sons and their families. To add to the tension, flights were delayed at layover points all across the Midwest because of tornadoes ravaging the land from the Great Plains down into Texas.

When we finally arrived in Pensacola, it was quite late. We rented a car and drove over the bay bridge to Pace, where Steven and Lauren lived. Everyone would be there except for Bob's daughter, who would arrive on Friday night, the day after next.

We drove to Steven and Lauren's neighborhood, and the moment we turned the corner and I saw their lovely house, my heart swelled with emotion. I truly thought it would burst.

For months I had envisioned this moment. I imagined my sons embracing Bob and welcoming him to the family. I couldn't wait to cook their favorite meals and play family games after dinner. In my head I heard laughter and saw camaraderie.

And now that moment had finally come.

We pulled into the driveway and went up to the house. Lauren greeted me warmly. Madison gave me a hug. Madelynn, Nick's wife, was pregnant and due to have their baby, a boy to be named Kobe, in a week. Six-year-old Madison was mothering Jasmine, Nick's daughter, almost a year old, and Lenah, Nadia's daughter, nine months old.

Steven came in from the backyard, gave me a hug and welcomed Bob. Nick was right behind him, but moving fast after Jasmine, yelling quick hellos as he ran by. Other friends were there visiting, and Nadia and Sean joined in the welcome.

I know my kids, as every mom knows her children. It was in the way they said hello. Instead of the absolute warmth and joy I expected and normally felt from my kids, I felt that their greetings were a bit standoffish.

We only stayed for an hour or so because we still had a forty-five minute drive to our hotel in Crest. There was a great deal of commotion, but I have to tell you that despite the slightly strange atmosphere, I was happy. I love having my children and grandchildren around me.

Finally Bob and I left. We had been up for nineteen hours straight. We checked into our hotel, which I'd chosen because it not only looked nice and clean, but was one of the known haunted hotels along the Florida route of haunted places.

We had the bridal suite, decorated with antique chairs and couches that looked older than antique. Gratefully, we dropped into bed and slept.

Thursday was a busy day. Bob and I ate breakfast and headed to downtown Crest to apply for our marriage license. Once that was accomplished we drove to the restaurant to meet with the owner and go over all the wedding plans for the upcoming Saturday.

The owner was a tremendous help. He showed us where the arbor would be placed on the dock overlooking the bay, and where the band would set up. He gave us a tour of the rooms where Bob and I would change clothes. He seemed almost as excited as we were. He invited us to have lunch. The seafood was delicious. Not fancy, but good.

Bob was exhausted, so I dropped him off at the hotel to rest. While he napped I drove to the florist to make sure everything would be ready for the ceremony. Then I went to the bakery to discuss the cake and make final arrangements for picking it up. Planning a wedding from a distance of three thousand miles had been nerve-wracking, so I was grateful that everything seemed to be falling smoothly into place.

When I got back to the hotel Bob had already finished his nap and taken a dip in the pool. Now he was showered and ready to go to Nick's for dinner. I got myself ready and off we went to Nick's home, only a mile from the hotel.

Nick and Madelyn owned a lovely two-story townhouse. Madelyn had a four-year-old son from her first marriage, a breathtakingly beautiful child with the face of an angel. He remembered me from the trip I'd made the year before. He climbed imme-diately into my lap and proceeded to tell me all about trucks.

Soon Steven and his family, Nadia and her family, and several of Steven and Nick's friends arrived. Nick and his wife had cooked a delicious Arabic meal; I was very proud of them.

Despite all this I should have seen the storm brew-ing, but I didn't. Maybe I didn't want to.

Denial.

Someone had brought wine for everyone to enjoy. Bob offered to open a bottle and serve everyone. Because some of the young people smoked, most of the adults hung out in the front yard. I stayed inside with the kids.

Shortly before Bob and I were due to leave, the babies were put down to sleep and I went outside to join the grownups. As I walked into the yard I could instantly tell that almost everyone there was a little drunk —except for Bob. He was *very* drunk.

He and I took a walk. I asked him to stop drinking. "I'm fine," he said, but agreed to stop. When we got back to the house the party was breaking up, so we said our goodnights and returned to our hotel.

The next day everyone was busy. The boys had to work, and I had to pick up the cake and go grocery shopping. I would be cooking a big meal for everyone that night.

After I shopped and got the cake, I dropped Bob off at the community pool in Lauren's parents' subdivision. The rest of the gang would be going swimming while I went on to Steven's home to drop off the cake and start cooking dinner. Everyone begged me to come swimming, and I promised I'd come back if I finished getting the meal together in time.

I must have brought the California weather with me, for the day was warm with a soft breeze instead of being larded with the normal hot, sticky humidity of Florida. I was excited when I wrapped my dinner preparations up in time to return to the pool. There, I found that the adults had been drinking a concoction Steven called Jungle Juice—a mixture of alcohols, juices and fruits.

I climbed into the water with Steven, Sean, Madison, Nadia, and Lenah—and my fiancé, who decided to show everyone just how hot he thought I was. He'd been drinking Jungle Juice, too, and he wrapped his arms around me and slipped his tongue in and out of my ear. My children looked disgusted. They'd never before seen me with anyone else except their father, who rarely if ever showed affection, especially in front of them.

I pulled away and told Bob to behave himself. He did his best, but Bob likes to do what Bob likes to do, especially if he doesn't believe what he's doing is wrong. To him, showing open affection for someone you love is fine.

He also doesn't believe in "steps." In Bob's opinion, if you marry someone who has children, then no matter how old the kids are, you love and support them as if they're your own offspring. Therefore Bob kept referring to my children and grandchildren as his own—and he expected me to feel the same way about his kids, especially after we were married.

I appreciated his feelings, and I knew he was sincere. I had no doubt that if my children ever needed or wanted anything, Bob would do his best to meet those needs and wants. That's the kind of man he is.

But my children were uncomfortable with him referring to them as his kids, or their children as his grandchildren. They asked him several times to please stop doing that, but he did not.

I tried to explain to him that the kids barely knew him, after all. I begged him to slow down and give them a chance to get to know him, and visa-versa. But Bob, full of love and Jungle Juice, did not or would not hear what I was saying.

Finally he and I left for the airport to pick up his daughter, Jennifer. We were both excited to see her—plus I hoped that if she were with us, Bob would feel more supported and less needy.

When we got back to the house, everyone had returned from the pool and was standing outside drinking wine and smoking. Since I neither drink nor smoke, I went inside to finish the cooking and spend time with the babies.

Once dinner was completed I asked everyone to gather around so I could lay out the details for the wedding the following day. But as I was explaining what I needed from everyone, I noticed that my children had become very quiet.

Finally Nick spoke. "We've talked it over," he said, looking me straight in the eye. "And we've decided we don't support you in marrying Bob."

I stared from one beloved face to the next. In Nick's eyes I saw nothing but resolve. In Steven's I saw resolve tainted with confusion of heart. In Nadia's I saw pain for me. In Lauren's I saw concern and fear, and in Sean's, the distress of a man who wished he wasn't witnessing the scene before him.

Bob's daughter Jennifer sat to one side, silently watching what was enfolding before her.

Bob was very quiet.

I was stunned.

"Steven?" I finally said. "Nadia? Do you agree with this?"

Steven hesitated. "Yes."

"I feel the way Nick does," Nadia said, "but Sean and I have discussed it, and even though we don't think marrying Bob is the right thing for you, we'll come to the wedding to show you support."

Again I looked from one face to the other. "But why do you feel this way? This is...tell me why you feel this way."

Nick leaned forward. "We shouldn't *have* to tell. But this is how strongly we feel about it, Mama: If you go through with this and marry Bob, we will never speak to you again, and you won't have anything to do with our families."

I just stared at him. I couldn't breathe.

"It's because we love you, Mom. Call it tough love; we're acting in your best interest."

I was appalled, embarrassed, shocked, humiliated. Not only for what my children were saying to me, but because they were saying it in front of their friends and Bob's daughter. For the first time in my life I felt ashamed of my kids: ashamed of them for treating me like this, and for subjecting Jennifer to such a lack of respect.

"I'm leaving," I said. "Bob and I are leaving together. Because that's where I belong now—with Bob."

My children begged me not to go, not with him. Their anguish made my heart break, but I wasn't sure what else to do apart from getting out of my son's home. I couldn't fathom what could have made my children feel so negatively about Bob that they would not support me or come to my wedding, and above all threaten to cut me off from my grandchildren. It just didn't make sense.

Truthfully, I concluded that my kids had simply made up their minds to not like Bob no matter what, and that explained their outrageous outbursts. They had never given Bob a chance. And for them to embarrass and humiliate me the way they had was more than I could tolerate.

As Bob, Jennifer and I drove back to the hotel, tears of embarrassment and humiliation rolled down my cheeks. I didn't know what to say. Bob returned silently to our room while I went to Jennifer's. She held me as I sobbed. I was humiliated by the horrid behavior of my children, especially since all I'd ever done was talk about how extraordinary and wonderful and special they were, and how eager I was for Jennifer to meet them.

The next morning I called my children. They asked me to come over, alone, so they could speak to me.

We gathered around the kitchen table in Steven's home: me, my kids, and all the in-laws except for Nick, who had to work until the afternoon, and Sean, who chose to sit in the living room.

One by one, my children and daughters-in-law told me why they did not want me to marry Bob.

Apparently, on Thursday while I was inside cooking and spending time with the grandchildren, I had been oblivious to what was transpiring outside. Bob had been drinking heavily, and when he drank he became, in my daughter-in-law Lauren's word, "creepy." Apparently he had massaged Lauren's neck, all the while telling her what a great mother she was. According to Lauren, Steven had wanted to kill Bob for putting his hands on her.

As for Madelyn and Nick, they were upset because Bob kept asking Madelyn if she wanted a glass of wine, as if he couldn't tell that she was pregnant enough to pop.

On top of all this, Bob—always very upfront about sharing his life—told my children and their friends about his daughter's first period, and how as a single dad he hadn't known how to explain it to her. "But she told me she already knew!"

Nor had they cared for how affectionate Bob had been with me in front of them. They accused us of acting like teenagers in love, which apparently completely disgusted them. God forbid their mother should be touched by anyone other than their father—and that had been years ago!

In the *piece de resistance*, as the French say, Bob kept telling my children that they were now *his* kids, and their children *his* grandchildren. He told them (over and over again) that he would be there for them, help and support them, because they were now *his* family. Apparently he repeated this so many times that even as my kids told me about it they seemed ready to explode.

"We told him over and over that we didn't want to be referred to as his kids," Nick said, "and that our children are not his grandchildren. He ignored us. We felt completely disrespected, Mom. He didn't care about our feelings; he only cared about his own."

Lauren leaned forward and said what might have been the most bizarre thing I'd heard in a bizarre day: "You should get back with Adam, Linda. He's changed. You two would be so right together."

All the way back to the hotel I pondered what I would say to Bob. I was emotionally exhausted, in shock, confused. How could things have gone so bad so quickly?

When I walked into our hotel room I found Jennifer lying on the couch. Bob approached me.

"What happened? Why were the kids so angry?"

Suddenly I felt calm. We sat down, and with no anger in my voice I listed my children's grievances.

Bob looked at me in astonishment, then turned questioningly toward his daughter.

"It's true, Dad," she said. "All of it. You were behaving so badly I told you to stop drinking, but it was too late. The damage had been done."

I stood up. "I need to make some phone calls," I said, and began to contact everyone necessary to cancel the wedding. Bob watched me, stricken.

"You're leaving me."

"I'm not leaving you, Bob. It's just that I'm not in any emotional state to marry you right now. I need time to figure things out."

One thing I already knew for sure: I would never be the wife of an alcoholic. Other than that, I was certain of nothing at all—not even that my relationship with Bob would survive. At any rate, this was no time for me to make quick decisions. Even though I was deeply in love with this man, I needed to process all my feelings and thoughts.

"I'm going to go back to Steven's," I said. "I told the kids I'd talk to them some more."

"You are leaving me," Bob cried. "Please, please don't—"

"No," I said. "We have to fly out the day after tomorrow so I can take care of the office while my brother's gone; in the meantime I need to spend time with my children and grandchildren. I need to work things out if I can."

"But—"

"Please don't call me constantly while I'm gone, Bob. I'll be back sometime tomorrow night." That made

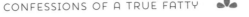

him look even more panicky. We both knew that we had to be packed and ready to drive to the airport at two a.m. to drop Jennifer off for her earlier flight.

I don't remember much about the rest of that afternoon. I do remember driving back to Nick's home that evening, and I remember Nick asking me what I had been thinking when I'd agreed to marry Bob. I remember him asking me if I was depressed, and how, without a thought, I said "Yes."

The word came out with the effortless speed of truth. Yes, I *was* depressed—and had been ever since Tommy passed away. Although I was also grateful for many things—the people in my life, losing two 245 pounds, meeting Bob, having a wonderful job—still, yes, I was depressed.

The life I was living was not the life I had envisioned for myself. My children lived too far away from me, and I needed them. In short, the happy exterior I presented to the world was a genuine yet terribly thin shell constraining an interior filled with turmoil. I was in love with Bob and had all the support in the world from my friends and much of my family—but with Tommy gone, part of me still felt as if it were missing. How much of me would remain if I lost my other children as well?

But I had never before felt so humiliated. Not even being forced to run back to my parents after the divorce had so completely destroyed my pride and self-worth as what my own offspring had done.

The next day Steven and I went out for lunch and, amazingly, had a pleasant meal. We avoided talking about the elephant in the room; we were content just to spend time together.

On the other hand, despite what I'd told Bob the day before, he kept texting and calling me. Sometimes I would answer long enough to beg him to let me have my day with my children; other times I did not answer at all.

Back at Steven's house, Lauren informed me that we had been invited to dinner at her mother's home. I respectfully declined—a social gathering was the last thing I wanted—and went to lie down for a while.

Nadia came in. "You *have* to go to Lauren's parent's," she said. "Lauren planned a surprise party for you."

A surprise party? Then I remembered: on top of everything else, the next day was my birthday. I looked at Nadia and realized there was no way I would get out of this party.

It didn't seem right. Was no one the least bit concerned with my feelings? But I knew Lauren was just trying to be sweet, and her parents, Miss Billie and Jimmy, were good people.

So of course I went.

Attendance consisted of my family members and several friends of Lauren's family. I put a smile on my face and did my best to appear fine when I was anything but. (FINE: Feelings In Need of Expression).

As I was admiring the birthday cake, I suddenly realized I'd seen it before. It was my wedding cake with the handmade white chocolate seashells removed and the layers redecorated with hot magenta and zebra ribbon.

Everyone seemed to be having a wonderful time. The succulent smells coming from the barbeque and smoker promised tender meats to be served shortly. I sat near my repurposed wedding cake trying to make chitchat while I wondered what Bob and Jennifer were doing. I was worried about Bob. And I was worried about my kids. But mostly I was worried about the way I felt.

Desolate.

When the food was ready, everyone gathered in the living room. There must have been over thirty people in there. We grabbed hands to say prayers

"Lord," Jimmy said, "we pray for Miss Linda that she will know the error of her ways, and to ask you to please open her mind to what her children are saying to her. Let her understand that sometimes we don't know what real love is until we let God come into our lives and show it to us."

Need I say that I wanted to die at that moment? I mean *really* die! Could I be any more humiliated? Was everyone taking pleasure in my pain? If not, why would they embarrass me this way?

Still, the party continued: the eating of dinner, the singing of "Happy Birthday," the cutting of the cake. I felt as if I was choking on every bite I swallowed.

Finally the time came to leave. Madelyn drove me back to the hotel.

What I didn't realize as I said good-bye to my sons was that that would be the last time they would speak to me.

Her appetite is non-existent. She orders breakfast but only plays with her food. The plate before her sits getting colder, its contents basically untouched.

Everyone else seems more concerned about their own feelings than hers. They seem to take no interest in what they're putting her through. She sits there with them, comforting them, trying to appease them. Can they not see HER pain, HER confusion, HER agony? Do they not care?

She prays silently: "God, why is this happening to me? Why can't I be allowed real happiness? Why am I being punished? You brought me this man to love and to be loved by. Why is that so difficult for others to support? Are you listening, God?"

She doubts God is listening. If he is, why doesn't he relieve her misery?

Apparently not even God is on her side. She feels all alone...again.

STUMBLING

CHAPTER 13

S he decides she can't die burdened with the feelings
she carries with her now. No: she must find a way
to solve her problems and escape from her pain.
Peace between herself and those she loves means more
to her than almost anything else.

Before she dies, she vows, she will regain her children's
love and respect. They will observe the love she shares
with Bob, and be happy for her. This revelation will take
time and patience to create, of course, but she knows
she can and will accomplish everything she wants to
accomplish.

But first she must stop feeling sorry for herself. Instead,
she must get angry. Sandie has always told her she needs
to get mad and stay mad long enough to make a difference. And Sandie is right.

She needs to finally feel her anger. Really feel it.

It's about fucking time.

I don't blame my children for what they feel. On that dreadful weekend Bob made a horrible impression on them. My kids got upset for themselves and frightened for me; they truly believed Bob was a threat to us all.

Worse, they felt that I had become a threat, too, simply by bringing a man they could not embrace into their lives. In their opinion, I had proven myself incapable of judging a man's character. They thought I had only connected with Bob because I was desperate to not be alone.

I was none of these things. I fell in love, and am still in love, with a good man who drank too much one weekend because he was nervous and intimidated, and alcohol took away his fears. But it also made him too affectionate, too desperate for acceptance, and as a result he acted the fool.

Although there's no excuse for Bob's behavior that weekend, the man my children responded to was not the man I fell in love with and chose to spend the rest of my life with. The Bob I knew was and is kind, loving, generous, and deeply caring. He wanted only to please. His biggest fault is wanting this so badly that sometimes when people meet him for the first time they feel he's trying too hard, that he's insincere.

But over time, as people get to know Bob they see the man I fell in love with; a very decent man who works incredibly hard to take care of his family. They see a man who puts other people first; a man who loves fully and will do anything for the people he loves.

But most of all they see how devoted he is to me, and how well-loved I am. They see him do his best every single day to make me happy.

That's why I love Bob like I have loved no other.

He's taught me about real love, long-lasting and devoted. He's shown me that I don't have to go it alone in life. He's not only at my side, he's in front of me if I need protecting, and behind me if I stumble and need support.

And there's been a lot of stumbling. At times I have to force myself to go to work because when I'm there I must act as if I don't have a care in the world. Then there are the day-to-day responsibilities I must attend to no matter how I feel.

And finally there's the fact that along the way I forgot everything I'd learned in weeks of classes about how to take care of myself after gastric by-pass surgery. I forgot that I'd gone under the knife to lose weight because I couldn't do it on my own. I did remember the many gifts of the surgery—getting rid of diabetes, having healthy blood pressure and boundless energy, feeling good about my body and myself, feeling grateful for finally having the life I believed I deserved. I took none of these things for granted then, or later.

Yet I still put the weight back on. My training didn't fail me; *I* failed me. I failed because when I tried to cope with my new problems I instead reverted to old, familiar habits. I forgot how to set boundaries. I ate and I ate. Not huge meals, and not a great deal at any one sitting—instead, I became a grazer. A grazer who made increasingly poor choices of what she put in her mouth.

At first I would bring cut-up vegetables and fruit to work with me to munch on. Then the cut-up vegetables and fruit became trail mix or nuts. Nuts became homemade trail mix—a combination of healthy nuts and a bag of M & Ms (king size so there will be more chocolate than nuts in the mix).

I internalized my pain.   My children's inability to trust my judgment, their ability to cut me out of their lives and those of my grandchildren so seemingly easily while being accepting of a father who was absent all the years they were growing up, caused emotional agony like none I had previously known. The choices my children made about me – not about Bob, but about me – demeaned me. And so I turned to the panacea I knew best: food.

Before my surgery I'd never been a grazer, but then I hadn't had my children cut me out of their lives yet, either. The last three years have been extremely stressful, and I admit that I have not handled things very well. The evidence—every single ounce of it—shows on my body.

When I returned from Florida it was torturous to have to face family, friends, and even patients who had earlier shared my joy of falling in love. My humiliation was a wound rubbed constantly raw by well-meaning people who loved and cared about me. For months I was asked about my wedding: why hadn't Bob and I married that weekend, as we were supposed to?

People didn't know, of course, that their questions about my non-wedding were immensely painful to me. How could I tell them that I hadn't gotten married because one day my fiancé drank too much and disrespected my children and me? How could I explain my embarrassment? The counter in a dental office is not exactly an appropriate place to share personal moments with patients.

So as my excuse for not marrying I used the slew of tornados that had ravaged the country that week, wreaking havoc with flight schedules. Not all my kids had been able to make it to Florida, I said, and I could never marry without all my children present.

Bob and I spent months talking, trying to see if we could salvage our relationship. He went to counseling, admitted he was an alcoholic, and did the work that proved, and continues to prove, how dedicated he is to our love.

I just wish my children would understand and accept the fact that I love both them *and* Bob. I want a relationship with everyone who matters to me.

It might seem strange to say this, especially since he was one cause of my humiliation, but thank God for Bob. He shows his love for me every single day. He still thinks I'm the most beautiful woman in the world, and our relationship is the one I've longed for my entire life. The weight I've gained since Florida has not changed anything between Bob and me. He faced his mistakes and fought for our relationship; he showed me that we could work together to overcome any problems that come our way.

Although I understand Bob's alcoholism—after all, I myself am a foodaholic—that doesn't mean I can or will accept alcoholism as a part of our life. He understands and agrees.

Perhaps because he is himself a former fatty (remember, he also had gastric bypass surgery), he knows all about using food to cope with difficulties. He tells me he simply doesn't see my excess weight. He loves me and appreciates me for who I am. Isn't that what we all yearn for?

I found that in Bob. He has nothing further to prove to me, my family members or my friends. He is worthy as a husband, a partner, and a family man; he would move mountains for me if he could.

I see what my children won't even consider: a man who recognized his weakness and addressed it. And while I know the healthiest reason for having done so would be for his own well-being, I also love that in part he did it for me, for our relationship. And it is both his strength in dealing with his drinking as well as his devotion to me that makes me love him all the more.

You might think that having all Bob's love and support would counter the pain of losing my children, but unfortunately that agony remains.

Somewhere along the line I lost myself. Well, it's time for me to fight for myself again. It's time for me to get out of this fat suit and into the body I want and desire – forever. It's time to stop living in the past.

For five years after the surgery I kept off the weight I'd lost. A year and a half after that I'd gained back 115 pounds of it. But in the subsequent year—and for the first time in my entire life—I did not gain any further weight. In fact, since then I've lost about fifteen more pounds, and kept it off.

The fact that I actually managed to do that, under the circumstances, shows me that I'm still willing to fight for myself.

I've taken responsibility for my part in the problems that sent me spiraling downward once again. I've apologized for the mistakes I made and reached out to my children countless times to try to resolve the issues between us. I even begged and pleaded with them—but was either denied or ignored. As a result, until recently I simply crumbled under the pressure, slipping deeper into the familiar, comforting ruts of depression and binge eating.

But now I've reached the point in my life where I know I've done all I can do to reconcile Bob and my children. I even sacrificed my pride—and gladly. Who cares about pride when you love someone, especially your own kids? Life is too short to be concerned with pride. We all must do our best to rectify, reach out, and take responsibility for the things we've done— and then move forward.

Gaining weight due to emotional eating accomplishes only one thing: it creates another problem to resolve. And it is a problem that (ironically) eats at you until any other problems you have become secondary to your obesity. When we binge eat, for a moment in time we go into denial, cushioned by the food we are taking in. But the question is, are we *really* comforted by the eating? Is compulsive eating a solution to anything at all, or just an unhealthy response to specific occurrences in our lives?

Once we come out of our food coma, reality inevitably sets in, along with guilt and self-disgust. While we're living in a binge state we avoid stepping on the scales. Why? Because we do not want to admit to what we're doing to our bodies. The scales display the evidence of our lack of commitment to ourselves, including our emotional well-being. Avoiding the scales keeps us safely in denial.

So, what is overeating really about? When we don't want to think about a problem, we simply create another problem to focus on. And that secondary problem is weight gain.

Let's get fat and become miserable!

Is this really the result we seek? Do we want to become more unhappy than we were to begin with? The answer is obvious, of course: no. Binge eating is not how we want to handle stressful situations. What we seek is the ability to take charge, to be in control. Feeling out of control is what makes us turn to food—the one constant we think we are controlling.

But in reality we're being controlled by the very substances we depend on to comfort us. We're in denial, shutting out the things that cause us pain, stress, or frustration; and we use eating to put us into a food coma, a fog of denial. Food, which is meant to nourish and enjoy, turns on us like an enemy when we binge eat.

I've spent my life trying to be a nice person, a person I'm proud of and like. I never understood that it's possible for a person to get angry and still be nice. Anger is a legitimate emotion; feeling it does not make us bad people.

Anger is a form of self-preservation. When we're attacked we do not have to accept the assault. We are not doormats to be stomped on or scuffed underfoot. Expressing anger can actually be constructive and conducive to bettering relationships and healthier living. What matters is how we *handle* our anger—and how we express it. We should be assertive, not aggressive. To be "assertive" is to declare oneself in a respectful manner, while to be "aggressive" is to attack your opponent, offering respect for neither the other person nor yourself.

She stands by her father's casket. Her Baba *is gone. This makes her sad, but not as sad as she feared she would be. It had pained her to see him suffering in the end, no longer the strong man, leader of the family, the man who solved everyone's problems—the man she had grown up with.*

No, this man lying in repose is far better off in God's care. It was his time, and she's grateful they had had far more years together than the family history had indicated they would. Most Misleh men passed in their fifties. Daddy made it to a few months short of eighty-two.

In her heart, she knows he lived a great life, a life lived on his own terms. Still, she will miss him terribly. He was always her rock, the one man she could depend on.

In the last few months her father barely spoke to her, at least in words. It seemed too much of an effort. She knew he hated being so disabled and needing so much care.

Two weeks before his passing, she was visiting him at Kaiser, leaning over the railing of his bed with her right hand folded over her left. Her daddy hadn't said anything to her in the hour she had been there, but suddenly he looked up.

"Where's the ring? Where's the ring?"

She looked at him, puzzled, and then realized he's referring to her engagement ring. She unfolds her hands and holds up her left hand."Daddy, are you talking about my ring? It's right here, Baba."

"Linda, marry him. Marry Bob. He is a good man. Promise me you won't wait. He is a good man."

"Don't worry, Baba. Don't worry...."

Two weeks later, most of her family, including aunts and uncles and cousins, gathered at his beside. He was dying. The nurse told them the end would probably come within the next twenty-four hours.

As they talked quietly around him, she swabbed his lips with a moisture stick and quietly prayed for him to let go. It was time.   Twenty minutes after they left the hospital, the phone call came. Her daddy, her Baba, was gone. They all hugged and held onto one another.

During the funeral everyone supports one another. She read her father's eulogy, which she also wrote. This incredible man came to this country with very little and died leaving a huge legacy. It is as if the end of an era has come to pass.

Her imperfect hero is gone. She only hopes she has not let him down in any way. Bob sometimes catches her quietly looking up at her father's picture and hears her whisper, "Hi, Baba."

She worries that in death her dad can see her and all her faults. Even as she deliberately eats harmful foods, she wonders if he witnesses her transgressions, and if he is angry with her.

Oh God, the guilt! The guilt! Even with him gone, she feels the guilt....

DON'T LET THE BACK LOBE RULE

CHAPTER 14

The face in the mirror is filled with anguish. The lies she's told herself are dead and gone. She's faced herself squarely, admitted the truth, stopped denying the tricks her mind has played on her.

But now a decision must be made. Is she going to continue to allow the past to submerge her in depression colored by the brief moments of joy she holds onto like lifelines? Or will she look upon the circumstances that brought her to today as a gift, a box wrapped in multi-colored paper and tied in a big magenta ribbon with a purple bow on top?

Of course, she has never been the type to see the world in a negative light. Always positive. Yet now, as she looks at her reflection and thinks about how she has handled her life so far, she wonders if the light and passion with which she faces events are simply ways to cover up a misperception of reality. If so, then everything she ever believed has been a pathetic falsehood.

Has a lifetime of cheerfulness been nothing but a wall of defense? Is her excess weight the result of a lifetime of pushing the truth deep down inside her? And is she now punishing herself for not living up to the ideals she so fervently holds?

She stares harder at her reflection. Looks herself squarely in the eyes—and the corners of her mouth soften into a smile. She knows her truth. She knows it better than anyone else.

She is a "Positive." She cherishes life, and feels that the life she's led is blessed. The people who know her love her. They love her for who she is, and although they do not care for her size, they bring that disapproval to her attention only out of concern for her health.

True, she's lived through a great deal of emotional pain. She's lost people she deeply loves, and is fighting for the respect of others who are still living. Someday she'll have that respect again—for her, there is no giving up on those she loves, or on life itself.

The blanket of fat she has so often bundled herself in is, in part, a defense mechanism. Well, the time has come to shed that blanket forever. Winter is over. Summer has arrived: the time to embrace the sun and allow its rays to penetrate her soul and recharge her inner light. That's what she lives for. That's what she deserves.

But she must also face some facts. She's too doggone hard on herself. She has to accept that she is not perfect. The image of perfection she's tried to adopt so others see her in the light she prefers is a falsehood she thrust upon herself. While those who know her best feel she has nothing to prove, she keeps pushing herself anyway. She has something to prove to herself.

The time has come to get out of her fat suit forever. No more excuses. No gimmicks, no surgery, no fads.

Commitment, dedication to the life she desires, and valuing her self-worth: these are the necessary first steps. No more self-judgment, no chastising herself. She is a Positive. She exemplifies a Positive.

Now she needs to take the beliefs she has always applied to others and apply them to herself. The time has come to put herself first.

The question is: Will she be able to do it this time...?

Am I all talk and no action? So far, I admit, I've been all talk. Well, some action. I've lost considerable weight on several occasions; I've had gastric bypass surgery; and now I've written a book confessing my food sins to the world. It takes guts to admit that you have the willpower of a moth around a light, except that in my case the light comes in the form of lasagna and chocolate. It also takes a bit of nerve to share all my dirty secrets about sneaking food, binge eating, and the fact that I am emotionally handicapped in some areas.

But what does all this really mean? As you read my story, do you hear echoes of your own? Do you feel the same frustration and guilt and anguish over being fat as I do? Like me, do you sneak food, or eat not because you're hungry but just because you *want* to eat?

Are you the person who takes care of everyone else before you take care of yourself? Let's say you've created a schedule that requires you to exercise every day at the same hour—would you give that time up if you received a last-minute request to cook dinner for your grown children, or babysit your grandchildren?

Do you tend to end up in charge of everything because you think you can do the job better than anyone else, or because you feel people will appreciate your contribution so much they'll view you in a better light? I call this "creating acceptance for yourself when you feel you have a shortcoming"—such as, say, being fat and feeling unattractive, and therefore seeking acceptance in other ways.

Do you define yourself by your size, or by your character? I know people who hate fat people. They can't stand being around them, and have absolutely no empathy for the issues that might drive a person to binge eat.

What about you? How do you judge *yourself*? Are you kind to yourself, or are you hateful? Does your weight hold you back from doing things you love, or trying things you've always wanted to try but can't because you're too heavy?

What, exactly, keeps you from losing weight and keeping it off?

Statistics say that 95 percent of people who lose weight gain it back. Only five percent reach their goal and keep the weight off. That sucks! Against odds like that, why bother losing weight in the first place?

Well, we bother because we have to. We must take care of our bodies—for reasons of health if nothing else. But let's be honest: most of us also abhor the way we feel in our own skins—and we hate all that excess skin as well. Ugh! Gross!

I lost my eighteen-year-old son when a freak virus attacked his heart. His death is one more reason for me to take care of myself. In taking care of my health—including my weight—I honor his short life; I show that I appreciate the fact I have a life to live. Why would I compromise my opportunity to live a fully healthy and blessed span of years? I certainly don't *want* to compromise that... yet I do.

Like all of us, I am human. Although I never intend to take life for granted, whenever I ignore my health (this goes for you, too) I'm basically thumbing my nose at life. We all think there will be another tomorrow, and another after that, and another—but sooner or later we're all wrong.

What would you do if you knew you had only ten years left before you passed away? Is there anything you want to see and do first? What if you couldn't do those things simply because you're too overweight?

Personally, I don't want to be the fat lady whose family has to buy an extra large casket to hoist her body into when she dies. I don't want the conversation at my gravesite to be along the lines of, "Wow, she needed twelve pallbearers instead of six, and even *they* were dying when they tried to lift her casket!"

Believe it or not, I've been to funerals where I've heard people behind me whispering expressions of this type about the person being buried. It's rude and disrespectful, of course—not only what's being said, but the fact that the women who were saying it presumably thought I couldn't overhear them. Or maybe they didn't care. The fact that I did overhear them only emphasizes how shameless those women were. It also taught me that people do talk. Even at an occasion as solemn as a funeral, people will cheerfully pick one another apart.

If imagining such a vision of your final legacy doesn't inspire you to lose weight, what will? I've spent most of my life being fat. Maybe some of us are just meant to be fat, right? Maybe we should just accept it and enjoy life the way it is, and the way we are.

I wish I could.

But for me, being overweight takes too much away from what I want out of life. My excess weight feels like the anchor of an aircraft carrier. It slows me down. I have too much energy to allow anything to slow me down. Which brings us back to the Big Questions: *Why am I so heavy? What's holding me back from losing weight and keeping it off?*

How about you? What's holding *you* back? Why can't you and I be the success stories?

Well, I say we can. The only thing stopping us is *us*. We all have excuses, reasons, emotional turmoil, boring times, stressful times, special occasions, holidays—again, reason after reason to not lose weight. But which are genuine issues and which are just excuses?

I recently had lunch with a friend—a new, dear and lovely friend who is also a psychotherapist. We were discussing my book. I shared with her much of the trauma of my life, including my obsession with food and my failure to lose weight and keep it off.

She looked at me with interest, and in a matter-of-fact tone told me my weight issues were not just psychological, but also physiological. My inability to lose weight was not really my fault; there are medical reasons why losing weight was so difficult for me.

But she added that this was by no means permission to give up. She explained that *candida* is sitting in my gut. What is *candida*? Yeast. When a person craves sugar or other carbs, it's because they have too much *candida* in their gut. Yeast feeds off sugar. When you eat sugar, the yeast devours it and creates more yeast, causing you to crave more sugar, and so on.

For the same reason, my friend also felt that I was misusing the word "addiction" when it came to food. Since my cravings are a medical condition, they are not a true addiction; they are a problem that needs to be treated medically.

That's what she told me...although I'm not sure I agree with the "addiction" part of the assessment.

I do, however, agree that those of us who struggle especially hard to lose weight have a serious medical problem. I also believe there is such a thing as an "addictive personality." Many people who've had gastric bypass surgery are warned about "addiction transference": the tendency to lose weight and stop overeating—only to then begin abusing alcohol, sex, or something else instead.

Like my new friend, some doctors recommend a high fat, high protein, low carb diet; or a gluten free diet; or a so-called Paleolithic diet. These regimens all focus on eliminating or at least diminishing sugar. I acknowledge that when I follow any such diet I do well. But it's important to know your own body and your own limits. On a low-carb diet my cravings for sugar and pasta greatly diminish...until I taste that first bit of cake, forkful of (sob) pasta, or handful of jelly beans. Like an alcoholic with booze, if I take just one bite I'm doomed. The moment I give in to these types of foods, I start gaining weight and have to start all over again to take it off.

It's all about paying attention to our bodies. But that means more than just recognizing which foods we need to avoid. We must also consider the emotional component of binge eating.

People like me use food in excess to fill emotional as well as physical needs. We have to learn what those emotional needs are and find ways to satisfy them that do not involve food. Call a friend; take a walk; slide into a bubble bath (if only I could so with my big fat ass), and so on. The truth is, we all know things we can do to help us get past those moments that drive us to eat. We just have to *do* them instead of taking the easy way out and heading for the refrigerator, cupboard, or back of the sock drawer.

My friend was astonished at the extent of my knowledge about weight loss. She said that the frontal lobe of my brain clearly understands why I should lose weight, and that analytically I know what I'm talking about when it comes to nutrition and weight loss. But as she also pointed out, it's the back lobe of the brain that controls appetite, emotions, and behavior and responses. In my case this back lobe is not connecting properly with the frontal lobe. It's *close* to doing so, she said—and once I get the lobes hooked together I will finally be able to overcome my obesity.

Then she asked me the 64-million dollar questions: *What's holding you back? What are you afraid of?*

I told her I'd asked myself the same things many times, in many different ways. What causes me to gain weight, and so much of it? And why do I then hold onto it?

A combination of factors is involved. Genetically, I was in trouble from birth. Then I started using food in a negative way during my childhood, especially my early teen years. Add to that the strong emotional ties I had to my dad, who I hero-worshipped and who I was always trying to please. The result was a formula for creating a fat kid who would turn into a fat adult unable to set boundaries and say "No" to anyone, including herself.

I'm not blaming my father for my weight gain. In the end, *I* chose to overeat. Still, I have learned—partly through writing this book—that my fixation on pleasing my parents, especially my father, and others in order to gain acceptance, led me into a lifelong habit of abusing food.

Only now, as a woman in my fifties, am I realizing how many expectations my father put on me to be the best I could be, to "be a leader not a follower," as he always said. Well, I ended up a leader amongst my peers, but a follower when it came to my father. His messages ingrained in me the need to always be a nice young lady, to be non-confrontational, to do what I was told. My father was the head of the household. He provided very well for us, yes—but in return, his family was there to serve him. This attitude wasn't his fault; his thinking was built on years of cultural messages thrust upon him, like those I myself clung to.

It took me most of my life to realize how much these mixed messages affected the way I handled myself. On the one hand, my father's immense loyalty to his family, always putting us first and providing well for us, is something I admire and have always strived to emulate. On the other hand, his dominance could be demeaning. I know that's not what he intended, but that was the effect. Although I never doubted that he loved me with his whole heart, *he* never doubted that his domineering ways were what were expected of a man. I didn't rebel against the domination because I figured, what's the use? In our house my father's word was law.

Yet the truth is that I *did* rebel—by feeding my teenage body up to a weight of 196 pounds. And then—on my own, at age fourteen— I showed my independence again by joining Weight Watchers and losing the excess weight. This reminds me that even when I feel dominated I have a strong spirit, an inner person who desires to be healthy and slender, and who is capable of reaching that goal.

I've been told that I need to admit to my anger at my dad for being so domineering; that until I allow myself to feel anger at my father I will not be able to let go of my weight.

But I cannot be angry with my dad. He doesn't deserve it. He made me feel loved and protected, and gave me a good life. When my first marriage disintegrated and I told him and my mother I wanted a divorce, they helped and supported me. *I* felt I had failed them; they never felt that way.

The truth is, I gained weight because I did not fight. I'm not talking about fighting against my father's strict ways, I'm talking about fighting for myself; believing in myself; taking care of myself. I gained weight because of choices I made and stories I chose to live in.

That's ironic because I've always been confident and assertive; I thought I believed in myself. And I do. It's just that I also consider myself to be a great nurturer; therefore, while I was convinced I could do anything I set my mind to (except perhaps for keeping weight off), I also always felt responsible for making sure everyone and everything else came first...which left me no time for myself.

Are you getting this? My belief systems—the ways I interpret the messages I receive from life—are based on the idea that everyone and everything else should receive my attention before I do. I've never felt that I deserve to take care of my own needs first.

And here's the kicker, the *why* of it: *If I put myself first, I'm letting down the people I care about.*

In addition, I felt that if I took care of everyone else first they would overlook my shortcomings, my failures, my weight. They would love me. I felt unworthy of other peoples' love unless I first made myself responsible for their happiness and comfort.

Again, this attitude came from my interpretation of the messages I received from my dad from early childhood on. He never intended for me to interpret the messages in this way, but I did. Call it immaturity, or a child wanting her parents' approval. The effect was the same.

What about my other parent, my mother?

She's always been amazing. She was the liaison between my dad and me. She's famous for saying, "Don't look back. Learn from your mistakes and move forward." She taught me about inner strength. I watched her handle difficult situations with power and dignity. When my father was too hard on us kids, my mother did her best to intervene on our behalf. Usually Dad won out, but my mom always gave him a good fight.

The down side of this was that she, too, put everyone else's needs before her own. So that's the message I got from her my whole life.

In addition, in Arabic culture there's also a strong taboo against shaming one's self or one's family.

Especially when it comes to protecting female virtue, everything seems to be *ayib*, shameful.

"Don't talk too long with a boy."

"Don't let even a bit of your stomach or back show when you reach for something."

"Don't reveal too much leg."

"Be sure to cover your knees with a towel so people cannot see up your dress while seated."

This shaming of women causes us tremendous frustration and guilt simply for being normal, healthy, sexual human beings. We are taught to suppress our feelings and desires, and that as women we should feel guilty for even having these very ordinary emotions.

We are also taught to serve our men and our families. I don't have a problem with that part of the culture except for one side-effect: even if a woman is dead on her feet after caring for others all day, we continue to push ourselves. Where is the consideration for *our* needs?

For those of you who think this is a women's lib thing, I'm here to tell you you're wrong. It's a common sense thing. If I can please the people in my life and cater to their needs, I'm happy to do so. But it makes no sense for me to provide for everyone else at the expense of my own health—especially when I'm tired or in pain from gratifying the whims of others.

But those are the expectations I carried into adulthood and my first marriage. I put Adam, his family, their negativity and their expectations—and of course the needs of my children—first, always. Which left very little time to put myself first, ever.

Adam's inability to show affection only intensified the messages that had been bored into me since childhood. If I could not earn the love and affection of my own husband, then I must be a poor excuse for a wife. I must be a failure.

But those things weren't true. I was a great wife and mother. The problems in my marriage stemmed from the same root: two people marrying one another for the wrong reasons. Despite the cultural heritage I shared with Adam and the treacherous, glowing image of my dream man standing at the foot of a grand staircase, in the end our personal belief systems were too far apart. I believed in him, but he did not believe in me. He was selfish. I never had his support.

Still, I was naïve enough to believe that with love we could overcome anything. This was not so. For whatever reasons, Adam stopped fighting for our marriage. Whether he lost interest in me when I started gaining weight or for some other reason, I don't know. But I do know this: I contributed to our dissolution of our marriage as well, by not fighting for myself.

I had a responsibility to Adam to take care of my body and my health. I failed in this area, and Adam couldn't handle it. He was unable to be supportive.

He simply stopped caring. Once again it comes back to me taking charge of myself first. Adam didn't like being married to a person who didn't take care of her body and who allowed others to use her as a doormat. Well, who would? It gets boring pretty fast, and respect is compromised.

In this book, this true fatty has made many confessions to you about my binge eating, about my life, about some very personal circumstances. But the truth is that none of the events I've described, either negative or positive, ever tied me down and forced tons of calories down my throat. *I* did that.

Whether I ate due to a physiological problem, or a psychological need to rebel, or to deal with emotional turmoil, my becoming a true fatty is the responsibility of only one person: me. *I'm* the one who hid food in clean, folded laundry so I could sneak it up to my room. *I'm* the one who sat in my car in a poorly-lit parking lot so I could stuff down chow from Taco Bell (which I don't even really like all that much; Taco Bell just happened to be open at that time of night!). *I'm* the one who hid Zingers between my chest and a magazine so I could sneak the cake in during my break and no one would tell me I shouldn't be eating stuff like that.

I'm the one who couldn't wait for KFC to open at ten thirty in the morning so I could order barbecue honey wings and mashed potatoes and gravy to scarf down while my kids were at school and my husband at work. *I'm* the one who stopped on a side street to indulge in a Philly cheesesteak before I went home to have dinner with my family. And *I'm* the one who bought Halloween mallow cream bats and pumpkins by the bag, not just once, but over and over again as soon as they popped up on the grocery store shelves. (I hid the bags in the zipper section of my purse or inside my makeup bag. I must have bought and devoured three bags before finally purchasing the one meant for everyone to enjoy for the holiday.)

Yes, I admit it: I am a true fatty. You have read my confessions. Along the way you might have cried with me, or laughed at me. I understand. Being a true fatty is not a condition others respect, nor is it easy to overcome. The addiction to sugar is strong and menacing, able to overtake sensibilities and destroy every wonderful moment afforded to those with a lean, healthy body.

But every day offers a new opportunity to transform our lives from the existence we have now into the adventure we deserve. I can't say "It's never too late" because it can be, of course. But right now it isn't; every day we are alive is an opportunity to change our patterns. So let's not waste the opportunity and take our lives for granted. We deserve the best life possible, and it's up to us to seek that life, to live it, and to share what we've learned with others so they, too, will strive for the best life based on our example. Don't be afraid to be that role model. But don't be too hard on yourself if you have days when you fail.

I figure that if I keep trying every single day to fight this battle, I will accomplish several things.

First, I will stop gaining weight.

Second, I will lose a few pounds and keep them off.

Third, I will show those who love me and are concerned for me that I can overcome any problem set before me; that I have the character to do so, or at least a strong enough sense of myself to keep trying. I can set the example.

In other words, I will never give up on myself.

We are not defined by our weight. We are defined by our character, by the respect we show others and the respect we show ourselves, and by the way we love. We are defined by our passion, our wisdom, our justice, our kindness, our empathy. Weight is only weight. It can be changed. Attaining outstanding character is far harder if you do not already possess it.

Thank you for allowing me to share my confessions with you. Please take away from this book the knowledge that there is someone who understands your pain and your battle. You are not alone. You and I share a common bond: we each want a healthy, lean, sexy, hot body. We are tired of jelly rolls of belly, saggy underarms, and front butts. No more front butts! We deserve to have healthy bodies, you and I.

And we owe it to ourselves to achieve that goal.

Compulsive overeating is something we do to ourselves. No messages from childhood, no rejection in adulthood, no external reason at all excuses us from hurting our bodies. When we get out of control it's because we let it happen. Staying strong, saying no, and getting our fat asses up off the couch are not easy tasks. But we have to do it, and we can do it together. We are doers and not the lazy stereotypes people think of when they think of fat people. We are strong. We are survivors.

I believe in us. I know we can unite and support one another. On good days we shall celebrate together. On bad days we shall share our burdens, lightening the load by reminding each other we are not alone. Although you and I might be part of the majority that struggles to lose weight and keep it off, at least we are not quitters.

I pray and put out into the universe that all true fatties who are seeking a healthy body at a healthy weight shall succeed in creating that body and keeping it for the rest of their lives. Although you and I might not be understood by those who do not struggle with food addiction, we stand together in knowing that we are remarkable people, strong in character, divine and beautiful, just as we are.

Thin or fat, take us as is.

She goes into the cupboards and throws out every unhealthy snack there: cookies, candy, cakes—all tossed. She opens the freezer and flings out the container of ice cream she had bought just the night before. The pizza rolls go next. How many times in her life has she done this, cleaned out her cabinets and fridge of unhealthy foods?

When it's over, the trashcan is full and heavy. Funny, she thinks: Imagine if I felt that same heaviness hanging on my body. How easy it is to take things for granted.

She sits at the kitchen table, grabs the weekly grocery store sale ads and goes through them, writing down the foods she needs to buy in order to start her diet. Healthy meats, low-sugar fruits, and fresh vegetables will be her new staples. No more foods containing sugar or flour.

She will not look at this new diet as deprivation. She will look at it as a choice she is making to enhance the well-being of her family and herself.

She walks to the cabinet that holds the family photo albums, pulls one out and goes through it page by page until she finds what she is looking for. Carefully, she pulls out one picture. There she is, sitting on a couch with her legs spread because she's too fat to sit with them closed. Her belly rests between her thighs, covering her private area with its massiveness.

She fastens this photo to the refrigerator door. It will be her reminder every time she wants to cheat. Beat the cheat, *she tells herself.*

Next she goes to the entertainment center and opens the drawer that holds her many exercise DVDs. Tomorrow morning, and every morning thereafter, she will make time to use these DVDs. And she will keep track of her progress.

She's on a mission. She knows it means she'll have to give up some things—heck, MANY things—that she's grown used to. But she can gladly give up foods she knows do not serve her well. Foods that can never taste good enough, or fulfill her emotional needs well enough, to be more important than her need to be strong within; to put her own needs first; to live the life she fervently desires.

She has finally found the life partner she always wanted. Fat or thin, her husband loves her with all his heart, and she thanks God for him every day. She also loves her children, and knows they love her. For this reason she's sure they will eventually come around and learn to accept that she's happy with her husband. They'll see how much love is shared between them, and how well he takes care of her.

As for her weight, every day she will strive to keep it under control. She's done it before, more than once, and she believes in herself enough to know she can do it again. She deserves the life she was meant to have, and will do whatever it takes to make that life happen. After all, the messages from her childhood and over fifty years of existence have made her into the person she is now. She likes that person. Apart from her weight, there's not much about herself she would care to change.

For her, life has not always been easy; sometimes it's been devastating. But she's remained strong. She's a survivor. She's a Positive, and believes in the goodness of the world no matter how naïve people consider her to be.

There's a reason she's gone through all the troubles that have come her way: she's meant to share her experiences so others can see that they, too, can overcome challenges in their lives. She can make a difference.

The next chapters of her life are yet to be written, but she knows they will be exciting and fun: the present time is HER time. She is taking responsibility for herself and her weight. She is putting her own needs first.

There will no doubt be further hardships to come, but she's confident she'll handle them with grace and dignity. Throughout her journey thus far she has learned enough about herself to take charge of her emotions, including those that govern her binge eating.

The life ahead of her is something she will embrace and cherish—like a terrific meal, but without the empty calories.

THE BEFORE AND AFTER SHOT

Food has always been a coping mechanism for me. Raised with food as the center of family gatherings, as a sign of affluence, as a treat for doing well, is it any wonder that like many of my generation I turned to it for comfort whenever life got uncomfortable, difficult, unmanageable? Is it any wonder that I became so severely overweight? But now I am ready to deal with my unhealthy dependence on food, and just as I invited you to join me in this journey through my life, I invite you to journey through your own and figure out what turned food into your drug of choice. Because while we may claim to like – to even love – food for food's sake, the fact is that if we are this overweight, our relationship with food is unhealthy.

When I began this book, I had intended it to open the discussion of overeating so that readers, seeing bits of themselves in me, would be inspired to take their own journey to well-being. And, I had also hoped that by the end of the writing of it I would be so much thinner that it would serve as a weight loss testimonial.

In every great weight loss testimonial we all want to see the before and after pictures. I had hoped I would be able to do just that in this book. I wanted badly to have a picture of myself at my heaviest; a picture of myself after the weight lost from bariatric surgery; a picture of myself after gaining one hundred and fifteen pounds back; and lastly, a picture of myself today, thin, toned, and sexy.

This is not the case. I have not lost the weight I gained. I have lost and gained and lost and gained so much over the last two years that right now I am pretty much the same as when I started to write this book. Does this make me a failure? Not in my mind.

This book is a journey. It is a journey for me, and it is one on which I have invited you along so that perhaps, in reading my story, you will learn a bit more about yourself and, at the end, we may all find success.

Through the process of writing this book, I have learned a great deal about myself. With you, I have shared truths about my passion for food. I have let you into the moments of deepest pain in my life: my divorce; the estrangement with my children; and the worst and deepest pain, the loss of my precious son, Tommy.

You are also privy to the good. The love and joy of my marriage to Bob; my love of, devotion to and need for my children; and the people I am privileged to know who care about me and my life. These blessings have rendered my weight problems and food addictions miniscule in comparison to what's in my bigger picture.

I wouldn't trade where I work for anything. Working alongside my brother and the people he employs is so satisfying. I consider these people I work with part of my family, and I love them.

The events that escalated my need to seek a source of comfort in an unhealthy way also brought me to who I am today and are an integral part of making me the person I am proud to be. So, while I would like to be thinner, I would not change who I am to be so.

My childhood may have been strict and restrictive in many ways, but I always felt deeply loved and supported. When I look back on the times spent with my family, I don't regret a moment of loss of freedom. Instead, I am grateful to my parents for wanting only the best for me. They taught me so much. I have my wisdom and devotion to those I love from my father. From my mother, I have an inner strength that is immeasurable; it has gotten me through dark times. And from her I have my kindness and compassion.

My ex-husband, now married again for the fourth time, has moved and is living near our children. To tell you that I am not envious that he is fortunate enough to live near them, to be able to see them daily if he chooses, and to share their lives with them, watching our grandchildren grow, would be a lie. He may not have been the best husband for me or the best father to his children, but I pray that instead of any of us focusing on the past, that instead we can focus on the new times ahead, and that new, good, and special memories emerge, diminishing the pain of the past, and glorifying the remainder of our lives.

I am happy to say that my children and I have come back together, reunited, strong and connected, with a love, respect, understanding, and compassion that can only make us better human beings.

I know my children love me. They have faced a great deal of tragedy. The divorce of the their parents, separation from one another, and the loss of a beloved brother is more than many people face as adults, let alone as children. Their animosity towards Bob and me and our marriage will change as they come to see how much love Bob and I share for one another and the solid marriage we have built. That one tragic humiliating weekend cannot and will not define us in the end.

I have raised strong hardworking and loving children. I am immensely proud of all of them. In time, I know they will come to an understanding that this separation between us was a moment for personal inner growth for us all. The love between us is too strong to allow us to step back from one another for too long.

As for me, I will never stop fighting to lose weight. More importantly, I will continue on my journey to optimal health. I hope to succeed before I am in the grave. Who knows?

I only can say that I know that any time we use anything to comfort us, to fulfill boredom, anger, hurt, and pain other than our own inner strength, we are letting ourselves down. There is no food, substance, or activity that will effectively fill emotional needs. Rather, it is in getting to the root of our problems or concerns and dealing with them that we access contentment. What's so wrong with feeling angry or sad or bored anyway? These are true human emotions. They deserve the same respect given to our times of joy and happiness. It is when we feel we need to be so strong, so good, so complacent for others that we suppress our needs and our feelings that we begin to self-destruct. And for many of us, that self-destruction comes in the form of overeating.

My dad in his old world ways, my ex-husband with his indifference to showing love, my children with the pain they feel I put them through, and my husband, Bob, with his need for recognition and acceptance, did not force me to binge eat. Food replaced facing, and facing down, the people I care so much about.

I was afraid they would love me less if I stood my ground more.

My daddy was my world. There isn't a day I don't miss him, talk to him feeling he can hear me. I am ever so grateful to him for his love for me and for the values he instilled in me.

My relationship with my ex-husband, Adam, is non-existent. He is the father of my children. I loved him while married to him and wished we could have found a way to make our marriage thrive, not only for the sake of our children, but for us as well. The pain our divorce caused our children is very hard to admit, but it is very real. I am sorry we put our children through it.

In my marriage to Adam, I never felt loved. Prior to our marriage he once said he did not believe in love. I guess that in my youth and naiveté, I thought I could change him by showing uncondi-tional love. I was wrong. Adam is who he is, and he has not changed.

Growing up feeling so loved, I expected to share love and be loved in marriage. That was not the case with Adam. His lack of love caused me to feel insecure, a feeling I never experienced prior to mar-riage to him. This new emotional territory and the uncertainty I felt triggered my need to seek solace. Rather than in the arms of another man, I found comfort in food.

I may have continued to use food in a self-destructive manner throughout the years, but I have proven to be far stronger than I give myself credit for. When Adam failed to financially contribute to the support of his children, I made up my mind that I didn't need him. I worked hard and built a good life for my children and me without his help.

When he neglected his children emotionally, I did my best to be father and mother to my kids. I never put him down to his children. I always gave him respect as their father. I felt doing anything less and disparaging their father would only hurt my children.

Today, he cannot hurt me unless he hurts my children. I have put him in the past. The relationship he has with his children is up to him to develop.

The pain I have felt in these last years separated from my sons has been agonizing. But regaining one hundred and fifteen pounds after accomplishing a loss of almost two hundred and fifty pounds is the fault of no one but me.

My sons had to come to terms with themselves, not with me. I respect their feelings, and I understand they thought they were doing what was best for them at the time. Today, I don't believe this to be the case. Perhaps I am wrong. For us to reunite meant letting go of the status quo and facing the fact that just maybe we had let the situation get out of hand.

Again, the problems I had in my family were not a green light to abuse my body. I have taken responsibility for my part in contributing to our family problems, as have my children, and we have found our way back to each other.

I chose to eat my pain instead of dealing with it. Simply, out of habit, and out of a lack of knowing and developing positive coping skills, I reverted back to how I knew best to deal with my turmoil. I ate.

I will tell you, I don't recommend it. Using food to self-medicate just doesn't work and is highly ineffective. Weight gain only makes us feel even more miserable. We have to learn to face the moments we fear in a manner that will not cause us more harm.

As for my confessions, well, all I can say is "Wow". I am some kind of crazy true fatty. Who in their right mind would confess to the world all their nasty, dirty, disgusting secrets about binge eating? I guess the answer to that one is me.

Don't judge me. We all have our demons. I know I have caught a few of you out there, like me, scarfing down fattening foods, eating alone in cars parked where we think no one can see us. I don't judge you. I feel you.

True fatties confess your food sins. If not to the world as I have done, then to your self. Admit your addiction to food. Admit you are a compulsive binge-eater. Face yourself and decide how you want to live the rest of your life.

We may never get to our goal weight, but I will be damned if I allow myself to go back to four hundred and thirty pounds.

Some day, I will write a before and after book. I will share my newfound ability to cope in positive and successful ways when faced with moments that would drive me and trigger me to over eat. Those pictures will be shared with you proclaiming that if I can do it, you can too. It is never too late to go from a before pic to the new and exciting after pic. We will prove to ourselves we can do anything we set our minds to if we want it badly enough.

I can't wait to share that moment with you. Till then, take me as I am. I am a true fatty that longs to be a true skinny, and I will work to make that goal my reality. This battle we have with food is not over until it is over, and it is a battle which, for the sake of those I love but mostly for my own sake, I intend to win.

Until we meet again...

DISCUSSION QUESTIONS

1. It is estimated that approximately sixty percent of Americans are overweight and that fifty percent of them are obese. And this is despite the multi-billion dollar diet and exercise industry. Why do you think so many Americans are overweight?

2. In what ways are women and men held back from living life fully because of their weight?

3. Do you think people who are overweight feel less deserving of enjoying certain experiences because of their size? What other emotions might someone who is overweight feel? In what ways might such feelings manifest themselves?

4. What insecurities do slender and overweight people share?

5. What do you see as the primary character or personality trait that separates slender from overweight people?

6. How likely are people to accept other people if they are overweight, even if they are otherwise personable, good looking, and professional? How unlikely?

7. In what ways does discrimination towards overweight people manifest?

8. In what ways does a person's being overweight inconvenience or impact others?

9. Does a person's size create an automatic opinion of that person in your mind before you have the opportunity to get to know them? When you see someone who is overweight walking down the street, do you find yourself judging him or her, possibly assuming they have no self-control, or perhaps think they should be doing something about their weight?

10. Have you ever been judged, discriminated against, or passed up due to something physical about you or your appearance? Or have you seen this happen to someone else? How did it make you feel?

11. What do you think has motivated Linda Misleh Wagner to speak openly about her addiction to food? Would you come clean about your addictions? If not, then why not?

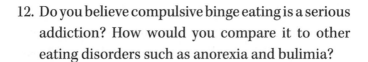

12. Do you believe compulsive binge eating is a serious addiction? How would you compare it to other eating disorders such as anorexia and bulimia?

13. Have you ever used food to comfort you? What kind of foods do you turn to?

14. How addicted are you to chocolate or sweets? What other kinds of food addictions are there?

15. Is emotional eating a true cause and reason for compulsive binge eating? Or is it an excuse? What might be roots of emotional eating?

16. What coping methods do you use when faced with emotional challenges?

17. Linda equates compulsive binge eating to addictions such as smoking, alcoholism, gambling, sex, and drugs. Do you agree with her assessment? Why or why not?

18. With statistics stating 95% of all people who diet will fail and/or regain their weight, how likely is Linda to succeed at losing weight? Do you believe in her determination? If not, then why don't you believe Linda can accomplish her goals?

19. Have you ever been challenged to overcome anything of great magnitude? What did you do to reach your goals? Have you maintained that goal? What other goals have you challenged yourself to meet?

20. If you have never had a weight problem, can you relate to Linda's problem with binge eating and using food to self-medicate?

21. Throughout the read, did you ever find yourself impatient with Linda and her weight-loss journey? When? Why?

22. Do you believe anyone can overcome any addiction, challenge, or hardship if they set their mind to doing so? What might get in the way of doing so? What do we need to be able to do so?

23. What do you think holds some people back from accomplishing their goals?

24. Do you have the courage to take a solid hard look at yourself and face areas of you or your life that should be addressed? What has held you back from addressing these issues in the past?

25. Linda Misleh Wagner believes she can do anything she truly sets her mind to doing? She believes you too can accomplish anything you set your mind to doing. Do you believe in yourself enough and do you know you can reach your goals, live a good healthy life, and fulfill your dreams? What changes do you want to make, and what are you doing today to start to make those changes?

Linda is determined to meet her weight loss goals, share her journey with you, and have plenty of before and after shots to share. E-mail Linda at linda@ lindamislehwagner.com and share your story. Start your own journey to fulfill your dreams and meet your personal goals. Let's do it together. She will e-mail you and keep in touch. We are not alone. We stand together.

If you would like Linda to visit your book group by phone, Skype, or in person, please contact Antoinette Kuritz at akuritz@strategiespr.com or 858-467-1978.

What was the genesis of your book? What made you decide to write it?

I was frustrated with weight gain. I first thought I would bring to light the frustration and demoralization of obesity by writing a funny self-deprecating book on the subject. And then I realized that by telling my story, I just might encourage others - and myself - to look at what in their life was making them binge.

You have been through a lot in your life. And you admittedly use food as a crutch. Why food? Why not smoking, drugs, etc? What led you to turn to food?

That's easy. In my youth food was equated with happiness, comfort, family, and celebration. It always had a positive connotation. Conversely, I wasn't allowed to smoke. And because of my upbringing, I couldn't imagine using drugs or alcohol or any other addictive substance. I didn't realize until much later in life how addicted to food I am, and it is only recently that I connected that I was binge eating to comfort myself. By the time I began gaining weight in my adulthood, I did begin to understand that I had an actual addiction to food and that I used food as a coping mechanism. And now that I recognize and understand my relationship with food, I am ready to work on it.

What coping mechanisms do you believe allow some people to deal with problems without turning to substance abuse? Why are some people more likely than others to seek comfort in food or other substances?

Some coping mechanisms are learned behavior. Families with a history of over indulging in food or people who have a history of alcoholism within the family are more likely to turn to these types of addictions. Genetics play into these types of behaviors also.

I honestly can't say what drives someone to choose say gambling over food, or sex, or drugs. I can only say they all share a common denominator. Addictions all feed an emotional need. For some reason, we don't feel we measure up to someone's perceived standards. They may even be our own standards.

What was the most formative lesson, positive or negative, of your childhood? How did that lesson impact the adult Linda?

Good and nice girls always take care of everyone and everything before they take care of themselves. And while I credit this lesson with my capacity for generosity and compassion, it also caused me to take too much onto my own shoulders and often fail to put my needs first when I should have.

Writing a book can often be cathartic. In what ways was it cathartic for you?

More than you can imagine. And it was scary divulging all my truths. But it forced me to look at myself, my life, and the psychological and emotional components of my addiction to food, and my use of food as a crutch.

You made great strides in overcoming your weight problem with your surgery, but you later gained a great deal of the weight back. What was the tipping point, and why were you still so vulnerable in this area?

There is comfort in reverting to old habits, especially when those habits are used for self-comfort.

Conversely, learning new habits takes effort. Learning to change the way we think takes work. When you feel you are under so much pressure to resolve issues in your life, the last thing you want to do is find a new way to cope. So when I hit my tipping point – the alienation of my children at a point in life that should have been my happiest – I simply reverted to old familiar habits. It is not something I would recommend.

What would be the first nugget of advice you would give to someone seeking to regain their health by losing weight?

Never give up. Even if you are not losing weight, keep trying to lose weight. I have not gained more weight because I have continued fighting to lose weight even on days I eat horribly. And now, a year into the fight, I am finally beginning to lose weight. And I am confident I can continue to do so.

You admittedly have tried every diet and every exercise tape out there. Why have they failed you? Why does the multi-billion dollar diet and exercise industry generally fail those who use it?

The diets and videos did not fail me. I failed myself. They all work. The problem is not the diet and exercise. It is our relationship with food, our mindset.

We have to fix the problem between the ears to solve our weight problem. And it is that problem between the ears that most diet and exercise programs fail to recognize.

What top three things do you believe it takes to overcome food addiction? Any addiction?

Commitment. Perseverance. And not coming down too hard on yourself if you have a bad day.

What role does patience play in losing weight and regaining our health?

We all want our diet and exercise programs to show immediate results. But we have to realize that we didn't gain all this weight in a week, or a month, or even several months, and chances are it will take a while to take it off and get back into shape. Be patient with your program and with yourself and celebrate the small steps because when taken together, they will make a huge difference.

You are obviously still strongly impacted by many of the events in your life and still vulnerable to your ex-husband. What does it take to extricate one's self from the hold others have on our sense of self?

The hold others have on us is because we care so much about the way we think things should be. A dear friend told me I hold onto the hurt. She was exactly right. At some point, we need to realize we cannot change other people's behavior, and we can only change the way we react. We allow into our lives what we choose to allow. I am not vulnerable to my ex-husband. I am vulnerable to the pain he inflicts onto my children. And yet, my children are grown and perfectly capable of dealing with their father and his shortfalls. We all have the capacity to keep certain things out of our sphere, to put them in perspective. We just have to gird ourselves and do so.

How important is sense-of-self to our overall well-being? Why?

I strongly feel I know who I am and what I am about. I am happy with who I am. I am unhappy with how I deal with emotions and situations. Knowing what we are about, what we stand for, and the type of people and life we want fulfils us. If you think poorly of yourself, you will attract negativity. We are all gifts with something genuine and wonderful to share. Find your strengths and spread them around to others. Find your weaknesses, and strive to do better, learn more, and grow. Above all, find what you like about yourself and focus on that while improving what you want to improve, all the while giving yourself the consideration you would give to others.

You seem determined to lose the weight and keep it off this time – to get healthy. Why will you make it?

Because I want health so badly. I know how great and wonderful I feel when I am at a healthy weight. I feel unstoppable, and beautiful, and young, and able. I will make it because I am not going to stop until I do make it. Because I am ready to put my essential needs first.

You went out on a limb sharing your story. What is the primary message you want readers to take from your book?

Our addictions do not define us. Our weight does not define us. These are symptoms of pain and unresolved hurt. Who we are is determined by what we do, how we give, and what we contribute to our life and the lives of those around us. I might be a true fatty, but my heart is what counts. In the end, we are measured by who we are and not by our size. And the best part is that when we can readily accept this, we just may be ready to get healthier.

ACKNOWLEDGEMENTS

Strategies Public Relations: The best day of the beginnings of my career was the day I presented my idea for my book to Antoinette Kuritz at the La Jolla Writers Conference. Antoinette asked to be my publicist. This incredible magnificent woman and her incredible team, Richard and Jared Kuritz, took me under their wing and helped me step by step through the process of producing a book.

Antoinette has been more than a publicist. She has been a Trojan mentor who has kept a watchful eye on every endeavor of the process. She has been instrumental in finding me the perfect editor, the right cover and interior designer, the distributor, any many other things that do not fall under the cap of a publicist. To say her company is a full service company guiding writers through the process would be an understatement.

Her attention to detail and her eye for recognizing the best direction to follow is perfection. Most importantly, Antoinette and her company have come to mean much to me. They have become cherished friends.

Mark Clements: I would like to thank my editor, Mark Clements. Mark had the wisdom to see the real story behind the story and encouraged me to follow its natural path. He believed in me and pushed me to not be afraid to express my truths without compromise of others and myself. Mark challenged me to dig deeper so I could produce a more fulfilling and meatier book.

GKS Creative: Thank you Gwyn for your artistry. The cover and interior are beautiful and express the perfect backdrop to the story.

Ameravant: To Ameravant, I thank you for the creation of my website. From the first moment I spoke to Monte, and then later to Michael, I was hooked. These gentlemen are in business to serve their clients well. They understood I knew nothing about the process of the website, and with ease, they guided me through the process.

Jennifer Wagner: Thank you so much, Jennifer, for the beautiful logos you helped me design for my website, LindaMislehWagner.com, home of the Future Former Fatty, and for my publishing house, MisWags Press. I put Jennifer under a very tight time constraint, and my girl, got the job done. She took my ideas and created logos that represent everything I could imagine. I am very grateful for your time and your beautiful talent.

My family: Thank you to my family, my mother, Susan, my brother, Anton, my sister, Judy, and my daughter, Nadia, my cousins, Hilda and Joanne. Their incredible support and encouragement has meant so much to me. They all have made me feel I could accomplish anything. I am so grateful for your support.

Sandra Ducheny O'Neill: My Sandie has been my greatest supporter since we were very small children. Her unfailing belief in me, her total support of everything I endeavor have meant so much. Her friendship is testament of a true love story between friends. I am forever blessed for having Sandie in my life. She always told me she knew I could accomplish my dreams.

My husband, Bob Wagner: My sweet husband has supported, encouraged, offered advice, and stood by me through so much. Bob, my love, if it weren't for your support and your courage knowing I was going to be as truthful as anyone could be, I could not have told my story. I thank you, sweetheart, for all you do to love and support me.